MYSTERIES
of the
JESUS PRAYER

MYSTERIES
of the
JESUS PRAYER

Experiencing the Presence of God and a Pilgrimage
to the Heart of an Ancient Spirituality

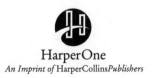

NORRIS J. CHUMLEY, Ph.D.

HarperOne
An Imprint of HarperCollins*Publishers*

HarperOne

All scripture quotations are from the Revised Standard Version of the Bible.

Grateful acknowledgment is given to the following photographers
for the use of their work in this publication: Norris J. Chumley,
Ahmed Farid, John Foster, Patrick F. Gallo, Dwight Grimm,
Todd Lester, and John A. McGuckin.

HarperCollins books may be purchased for educational, business, or
sales promotional use. For information, please write: Special Markets Department,
HarperCollins Publishers, 10 East 53rd Street, New York, NY 10022.

HarperCollins website: http://www.harpercollins.com

HarperCollins®, 📖®, and HarperOne™
are trademarks of HarperCollins Publishers

FIRST EDITION

Designed by Ralph Fowler

Library of Congress Cataloging-in-Publication Data is available upon request.

ISBN 978–0–06–187417–8

11 12 13 14 15   RRD (H)   10 9 8 7 6 5 4 3 2 1

This book is dedicated to Jesus Christ,

and the likeness of him in all of us.

Contents

Foreword

IT IS WITH SPIRITUAL DELIGHT that we welcome and introduce this book on the living tradition and profound *Mysteries of the Jesus Prayer,* as preserved and practiced in Orthodox monasteries today throughout the world.

Many centuries ago, in fourth-century Constantinople, a monastery was established, which came to be known as the community of the "sleepless ones" (or *Akoimetoi*), since worship and contemplation continued there without interruption all day and night. Orthodox Christian monasteries have always aspired to be places of fervent and ceaseless prayer. People have visited such places in order to discover men and women of prayer and holiness. And the Jesus Prayer has become established in Orthodox Christianity as a unique symbol of intense and unceasing prayer. It is the silent prayer of the heart, the living seed of all spiritual life and theological thought.

Nonetheless, for St. Basil the Great in fourth-century Cappadocia, the monastic way is nothing more than "the life according to the Gospel." Everyone is invited to respond to the call of Christ; monks and nuns simply realize this goal in a unique way. Similarly, the Jesus Prayer has its roots in Scripture, particularly in the exhortation of St. Paul to "pray without ceasing" (1 Thess. 5:17) Thus, the mysteries of the Jesus Prayer are not the privilege of a few, but the vocation of all.

Moreover, prayer is a relationship word; it can never be thought of in abstraction, isolated from others or from God. Unfortunately, we have reduced prayer to a private act, an occasion for selfish concern or complaint. Yet prayer is never exclusive or divisive; it is inclusive and caring. Authentic prayer is never self-serving or self-complacent; it involves a sense of compassion for all people and all creation.

The whole Orthodox understanding, discipline, and teaching about prayer may be condensed into the short formula commonly known as the "Jesus Prayer." It is a prayer solemnized in the classic writings of *The Philokalia* and popularized through such contemporary works as *The Way of a Pilgrim,* an anonymous nineteenth-century story of a Russian wanderer, and J. D. Salinger's mid-twentieth-century stories from *The New Yorker,* published separately under the title *Franny and Zooey.*

"Lord Jesus Christ, Son of God, have mercy on me." This brief prayer is a simple prayer and not a complicated exercise. The Jesus Prayer can be used by everyone as a concise, arrow-prayer that leads directly from our heart to the heart of God via the heart of the world. It is the realization—beyond the recitation of conventional prayers—of the power of silence. For when prayer culminates in silence, we awaken to new awareness. Then, prayer becomes a way of noticing more clearly and responding more effectively to the world within us and around us.

May this book open up the blessings and "mysteries of the Jesus Prayer" to a wide number and range of people.

—BARTHOLOMEW
Archbishop of Constantinople, New Rome,
and Ecumenical Patriarch

MYSTERIES
of the
JESUS PRAYER

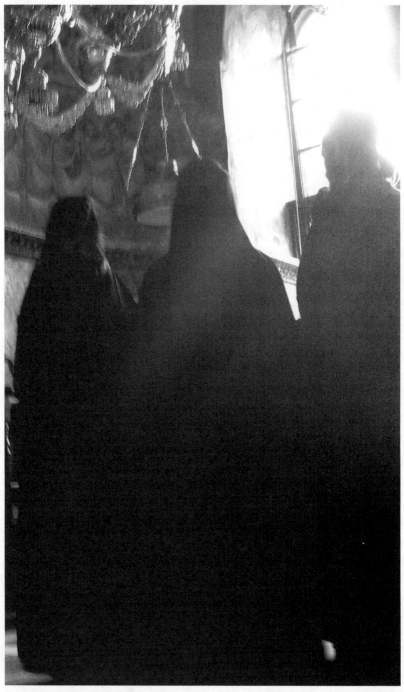

Introduction

L YING ON MY DESK within easy reach is a small circlet of leather with a leather cross dangling from it. Woven into the circlet are one hundred wooden dowels. This object is a *lestovka* (or "ladder"), the traditional prayer rope of Ukrainian and Russian Orthodox Christians. It was given to me by Father Paisij, a monk and deacon of the St. Jonas Monastery in Kiev, Ukraine. My friend Father John McGuckin tells me that my *lestovka* is very old, very rare.

I keep this treasured prayer rope always at hand, and often when I say the Jesus Prayer, my fingers move across the dowels and I remember Father Paisij and think of the countless other men of God who have prayed with this humble yet beautiful object.

A moment ago I mentioned the Jesus Prayer. It's likely that you aren't familiar with it. Few people in our part of the world have ever heard of it. In fact, it was to bring the Jesus Prayer to the West that Father John and I made the film *Mysteries of the Jesus Prayer* and wrote this companion volume.

The Jesus Prayer goes like this:

Lord Jesus Christ, Son of God, have mercy on me, a sinner.

Opposite: The Vatopedi fathers on Mount Athos sing the Holy Liturgy as the thousand-year-old *katholikon* (or primary church) is illuminated by the morning's first light.

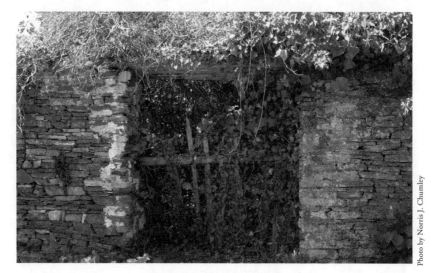

Photo by Norris J. Chumley

An ancient gate on Mount Athos, near a skete (hermitage)
where hermits reside and pray.

For at least 1,700 years this seemingly simple prayer has been the
cornerstone of the spiritual life of countless monks and nuns of the
Eastern Church. Yet outside the walls of their monasteries and convents, very few Christians—even those within the Eastern tradition—have ever heard of this prayer or experienced its power to touch
the soul and transform one's life.

In *Mysteries of the Jesus Prayer* Father John and I have done our best
to *de*mystify this ancient prayer, taking it out of remote monasteries
and desert caves and into the lives of millions of believers who are
yearning for the peace and reassurance that come from forming a
deeper connection with God.

Both the film and this book are the fruit of a spiritual quest undertaken over the last eight years, a travelogue of the heart and mind that
Father John and I made to document our search for ancient wisdom
and spiritual practices that have been fundamental to the day-to-day
life of Orthodox Christian monks and nuns. In our conversations
with these holy, dedicated men and women, they revealed a secret to
us that mystics have known for centuries: God is found in silence and
through the constant interior repetition of the Jesus Prayer.

Introduction

No one knows who composed the Jesus Prayer. We hear echoes of it in various verses in the Gospels. Some of the monks we met believe that the Jesus Prayer originated with Jesus Christ's apostles. That is possible, but we simply don't have conclusive evidence. In any case, it is not the *age* of the prayer that is important, but its *power*.

As you read further, you'll find that we have drawn upon classic texts of great saints and mystics who wrote about the Jesus Prayer, but your more immediate guides will be contemporary monks and nuns, bishops, and abbots and abbesses who know the mysterious power of the Jesus Prayer through personal experience. These holy men and women offered their full cooperation with this project; as a result, for the first time these private mystical practices can be revealed and shared with mass audiences.

The Jesus Prayer was the wellspring of Christianity's first mystical tradition. In the second century its power was discovered by ascetics and hermits in the deserts of Egypt and Syria. As Christianity spread across eastern Europe, it carried with it the mystical practices of the Desert Fathers and Mothers. To this day the constant recitation of and

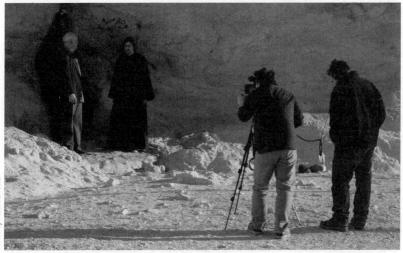

Photo by Ahmed Farid

Filming at St. Antony's cave, high above his monastery, near Al-Zaafarana on the Red Sea in Egypt. Our directors of photography, Patrick Gallo and Dwight Grimm, record our comments.

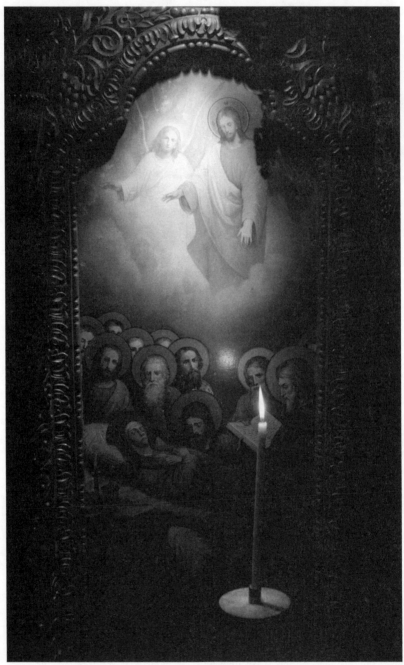

Chapel icon in St. Ana's Monastery, Rohia, Romania. This icon is tucked away in a side wing of the underground chapel under the main church.

Photo by John A. McGuckin

meditation upon the Jesus Prayer remains a central part of the spiritual life within the monasteries and convents of Eastern Christianity.

To find these master contemporary spiritual teachers, Father John and I traveled throughout the early Christian world—to St. Antony's Monastery in the Egyptian desert and St. Catherine's Monastery on Mount Sinai, to convents in Transylvania, and to monasteries in Russia, in Ukraine, and on Mount Athos in Greece. In all of these places we were overwhelmed by the generosity of the monks and nuns who were eager to share with us—and with you—how to move through the various stages of prayer: from the basic prayer of petition, to a prayer of praise, to the goal of every mystic—a direct experience of being in the presence of God.

Father John and I know from personal experience that the Jesus Prayer has the power to still the clamor and distractions of the world, to offer calm and reassurance to those who feel agitated and anxious, and to eliminate the illusion that a vast, unbridgeable gulf separates us from God. The Jesus Prayer purges the isolation and loneliness of modern life, revives the interior life that has been deadened by confusion and unhappiness, and fills the heart, mind, and spirit with the realization that God exists and that he wills for us to be in continuous communion with him.

I thank you for joining us on this spiritual quest, and I pray that you will experience in a profound way the power of the Jesus Prayer to touch the soul and change lives.

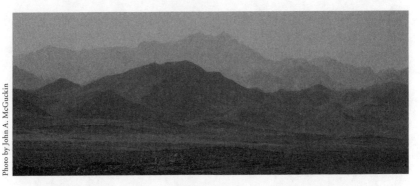

Photo by John A. McGuckin

The Egyptian desert, near Al-Qalzam Mountain. This was what St. Antony likely saw for forty-six years outside his mountain cave.

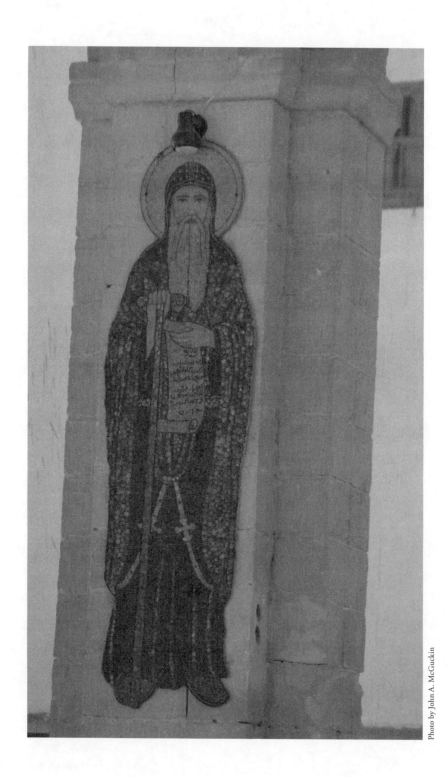

I

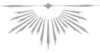

The Power of the Jesus Prayer

Lord Jesus Christ, Son of God, have mercy on me, a sinner.

T HIS BOOK IS A TRAVELOGUE of the heart, and the mind, and the feet.

It was conceived eight years ago during a conversation about the power and mystery of the Jesus Prayer between Father John McGuckin, a priest of the Orthodox Church, and me, a student of theology and spiritual seeker. During that discussion it came to us that we ought to imitate the example of other seekers and go on pilgrimage to call upon monks and nuns of great holiness, wisdom, and spiritual insight who could reveal to us the treasures of the Jesus Prayer and help us make it truly the prayer of our hearts.

We decided to model our pilgrimage on a journey undertaken 1,400 years ago by two other seekers, St. John Moschos (died c. 619), a monk from Judea, and his friend, protégé, and fellow monastic St. Sophronius (died c. 639). As a young man John had entered the Monastery of St. Theodosios outside Bethlehem—a monastery built, it was said, over a cave where the Magi rested on their star-led quest to find the Christ Child. About the year 568 John, in pursuit of a

---

Opposite: Mosaic of St. Antony on a pillar just inside the entrance of the monastery.

stricter form of the monastic life, transferred to the Monastery of St. Chariton in the Judean desert. There he met Sophronius. After ten years at St. Chariton the two friends decided to travel to Egypt and the Sinai Peninsula in search of the wisest, holiest monks, hoping that these holy men could teach them how to immerse themselves completely in the love of God.

"God Alone"

The word "monasticism" comes from the Greek word *monos,* which means "to dwell alone." And in fact the first monks did dwell alone, living as hermits in remote corners of the Roman Empire. Tradition tells us that St. Paul the Hermit (c. 230–343) was the first of these Christian solitaries. He was an Egyptian, the son of a well-to-do family. At age twenty-two, to escape the anti-Christian persecution begun by the Roman emperor Decius, Paul traveled deep into the Theban Desert, where he found an empty cave. He lived there all alone for the next ninety years.

It's often said that the first hermits went into the desert to escape the vices of the pagan world, but that's only part of the story. The hermit, the monk, the nun—each of these individuals desires to love God above all things, and so he or she puts aside every obstacle that interferes with loving God: wealth, status, career, family, friends. This concept is summed up in one of the most famous mottoes of monastic life: "God alone."

By the mid-fourth century, there were thousands of hermits scattered across the wastelands of the Near East, living in caves, huts, even empty tombs. Sometimes they would gather near the cave of an especially holy hermit, forming a kind of loose community. That designated hermit would take on the role of informal abbot, directing the spiritual formation of his disciples. Generally in these early "monasteries," each member lived, worked, and prayed alone, coming together with his brothers only for the Eucharist (or the Holy Sacrifice of the Mass as it is known in Catholicism, the Divine Liturgy as it is known in the East). Such was the case with St. Antony of the Desert.

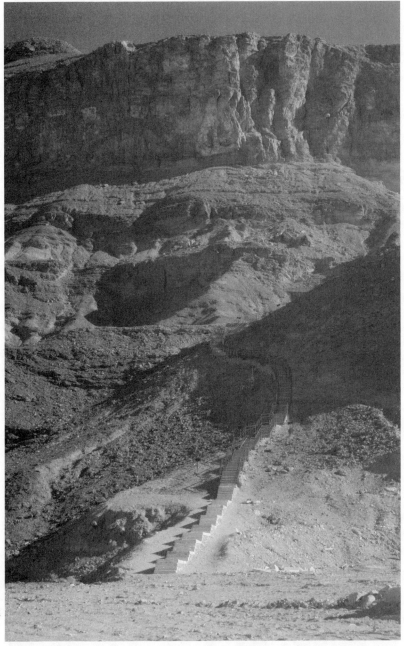

Photo by John A. McGuckin

The monks installed over 1,100 steps up the cliff from the monastery to St. Antony's cave. It took us about an hour to traverse the almost 300-meter climb. All along the way there are signs with psalms written on them in various languages.

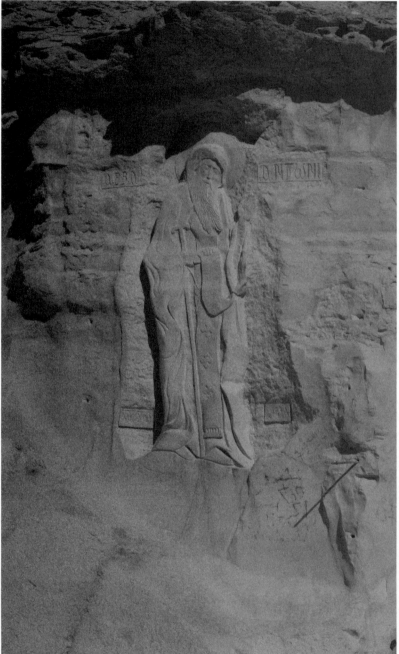

Around the corner from the monastery is this gigantic stone carving of St. Antony on the side of a mountain. Pilgrims encounter it on the way to the saint's cave home.

So many hermits sought his spiritual counsel that in 305 he gave up, reluctantly, his solitary life of prayer and penance and established the first monastery at what is now Deir el-Memum in Egypt. Five or six years later he moved to the desert that lies between the Nile and the Red Sea. There he lived in a cave in a cliff overlooking the Red Sea. After the death of St. Antony in 356, a monastery named Deir Mar Antonios was established in his memory near the foot of the cliff where he spent the last years of his life. That monastery is still in existence today—in fact, Father John and I visited it.

Within a century after St. Antony's death, monasticism had spread from Egypt throughout the East, across the Mediterranean to Europe, and as far west as Ireland. Monastic rituals, customs, and even day-to-day schedules varied from one community to the next, but in one thing the monks were united—their desire to grow closer to God through constant prayer.

The Spiritual Treasure of the East

The fruit of Sts. John and Sophronius's pilgrimage is the classic text *The Spiritual Meadow,* a collection of the sacred sayings, stories, and parables of the holy monks the two friends met during their wanderings in the deserts of the Near East. John, who wrote the book, dedicated it to Sophronius, saying that the wisdom they acquired from the holy men was like a meadow full of different wildflowers, one more beautiful than the next. "From among these I have plucked the finest flowers of the unmown meadow," John writes, "and worked them into a crown which I now offer to you, most faithful child; and through you, to the world at large."

Father John and I, like John and Sophronius, left our homes and wandered to far-off places in search of holy wisdom—but ours was a quest with a difference. While John and Sophronius collected a kind of grab bag of monastic teachings, we had a single goal in mind: we wanted to delve into the life-transforming power of the Jesus Prayer and make this spiritual treasure of the East known, loved, and practiced in the West.

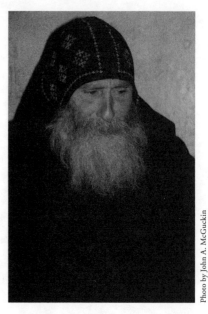

Father Lazarus, the starets (spiritual
leader) of St. Antony's Monastery, made
a rare exception to be photographed. He
spends most of his time secluded in his
mountainside cave above the monastery.

Our journey led us to caves in the Egyptian desert, to white-
washed island chapels in the Aegean, to catacombs in Kiev, to convents hidden away in the forests of Romania. Everywhere we went we
met profound teachers—men and women—who assured us that true
peace is possible, peace within ourselves and peace between individuals. These monks and nuns knew from personal experience that peace
is not an abstraction, but a living reality, and they taught us that the
first step toward peace is entrusting your life in every way to God.
How is this accomplished? First, through surrender—in other words,
by putting ego aside and making communion with God the primary
purpose of your life. These holy men and women were trying to put
into practice an ideal that the Spanish mystic St. John of the Cross
articulated in his *Spiritual Maxims* nearly 500 years ago: "Live in the
world as if only God and you were in it; then your heart will never be
made captive by any earthly thing."

The next step is to set aside a regular time when you will shut off the
phone, the computer, the television, and the radio and in the stillness
give yourself up to silent prayer and contemplation. Few of us can with-

draw completely from the world, but that is not a stumbling block. By all means, fulfill your obligations to family, friends, work, and neighborhood, but make your actions an extension of your prayer life.

What happens in the lives of the monks and nuns is that all human-made concepts and reasoning are surrendered to God. This emptying offers room for divine inspiration and spiritual thoughts to enter the mind. St. Gregory of Sinai described this in the fourteenth century: "Prayer is God, who works all things in men." It is God doing the work of silence and prayer, "no longer I . . . but Christ who lives in me" (Gal. 2:20). John the Baptist said of Christ, "He must increase, but I must decrease" (John 3:30). The purpose of the work of the monastics is to let God fully exist inwardly, and to let God control their lives accordingly. The method of silence is nothing like emptiness or inactivity; on the contrary, it is a full life of unity with God in divine action and purpose, listening for God in every aspect of internal and external life.

The vigilant waiting in silence is so that God's presence may be felt and God's directives followed. "Be still, and know that I am God" (Ps. 46:10). The monk or nun enters into the innermost hidden, quiet realm of herself and in silence and pure stillness finds God waiting.

In the East for nearly 2,000 years the devout and the spiritually enlightened have drawn upon the power of the Jesus Prayer to experience continually a direct mystical union with God. Having originated as early as the time of the apostles and developed from the fifth to the fourteenth centuries, the Jesus Prayer provides a true and complete method of peace, liberation, and salvation. The purpose of our journey, the goal of this book, is to bring to the Western world an ancient prayer that can liberate us from fear and anxiety, help us to discover peace and happiness, and enable us to live each moment in the loving presence of God.

A Spiritual Paradise

No one knows the name of the Christian who composed the Jesus Prayer, but it is likely that the petition reaches back to the origins of

Christianity itself. In the Gospel of St. Luke we read of a blind man sitting by the side of the Jericho road. He is aware that a throng of people are passing by, and when someone in the crowd tells him that Jesus of Nazareth is coming, the blind man lifts up his voice and cries, "Jesus, Son of David, have mercy on me!" (Luke 18:38). It sounds very close to the Jesus Prayer; and if that cry of the blind man is the source, then the Jesus Prayer, along with the Lord's Prayer and the Hail Mary, is rooted in scripture and is just as ancient.

When we were in Romania, Archbishop Justinian Chira Maramureşeanul of Baia Mare told us that he believes the Jesus Prayer originated with Christ's apostles. According to the archbishop, "[After] the ascension of Christ to heaven, the apostles stayed alone and they started day and night to say this prayer—Jesus Christ, Son of God, have mercy. It was the only way to keep contact with the One who had ascended to heaven through thought, image, and sound."

The Jesus Prayer as we know it—"Lord Jesus Christ, Son of God, have mercy on me, a sinner"—dates at least to the second century. It may have been part of the prayer life of St. Paul the Hermit. It was certainly part of the prayer life of St. Antony of the Desert and the men who came together to found the first Christian monastery.

To this day monasteries tend to be located in out-of-the-way places, because centuries of experience have taught the holy men and women who populate them that only in the stillness of such isolated spots can they silence their own unruly passions and hear the voice of God. Isolated from the chatter, cares, and busyness of the world, they hope to find ecstasy beyond the physical pleasures of sexuality, wisdom more profound than any philosophy, a connection deeper and more permanent than that of any friendship. The first hermits, monks, and nuns went into the desert to discover a spiritual paradise, and they found that they could reach that paradise by practicing what St. Antony called "the prayer of quiet."

But living in a quiet place is not enough. St. Antony taught his monks to develop *interior* silence—that is, to focus the mind and heart on God, not letting their interior silence be hijacked by impulses, random thoughts, or even memories, all of which create their

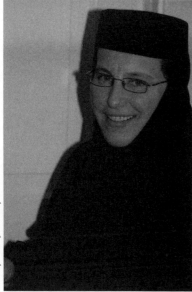

Photo by Norris J. Chumley

Sister Josephina Giosanu, abbess of
Văratec Monastery in Romania. See the
joy and warmth of God in her smile?

own kind of internal "noise" that distracts the seeker from the thing
he or she desires above all: connection with God. The silence that
St. Antony recommended is not the absence of sound, such as we
would encounter standing all alone in an empty room; rather, it is
a silence with a purpose. We choose to keep still in order to become
increasingly aware of the presence of God.

St. Antony himself taught his monks how to achieve interior silence, and so began a spiritual mentor-protégé system that survives
to this day. The prayer the masters have always recommended—and
still recommend—to the novices is, "Lord Jesus Christ, Son of God,
have mercy on me, a sinner." But the saints knew that the Jesus Prayer
alone would not be enough: first and foremost they all needed the
grace of God, because no one can become holy without it; furthermore, they needed the Holy Mysteries—the Eucharist, which the
monks and nuns received at the Divine Liturgy, the pinnacle of prayer
in the Eastern Church. Fed with the Eucharist, strengthened with
God's grace, the monk or nun was ready to keep still and be open to
an experience of God.

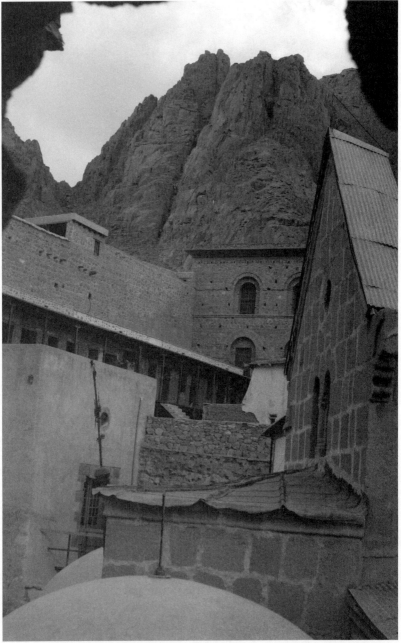

Photo by John A. McGuckin

Monks' cells at St. Catherine's Monastery, with part of Mount Sinai in the background. These are the ancient rooms where the fathers pray through the night, getting only a few hours of sleep.

The Geography of the Heart

In addition to being known as "the prayer of quiet," the Jesus Prayer is also commonly referred to as "the prayer of the heart." St. Theophan the Recluse (1815–1894), a Russian master of the spiritual life, declared, "To pray is to stand before God with the mind in the heart." What can that mean, to have "the mind in the heart"? As children of a rational, scientific age, we know the heart as a muscle that pumps blood through the body. The saints knew that basic fact, too, but they also viewed the heart metaphorically. St. Macarius the Great (c. 300–c. 390), an Egyptian abbot who directed the spiritual life of thousands of monks, tells us, "The heart is but a small vessel; and yet dragons and lions are there, and there poisonous creatures and all the treasures of wickedness; rough, uneven paths are there, and gaping chasms. There likewise is God, there are the angels, the heavenly cities and the treasures of grace; all things are there." The heart, then, is a conflicted place, an inner chamber where we conceal our worst impulses, but also an inner temple where we commune with God. The mind, on the other hand, is the seat of skepticism, uncertainty, and doubt. To thrust the mind into the heart as St. Theophan recommends is to drown our doubts in the boundless love of God. And constant prayer, particularly the Jesus Prayer, expels the vices from the heart so that Jesus Christ may enter and make it entirely his own.

The Pitfalls

There was a period when Father John and I wondered if perhaps the Jesus Prayer had not been intended for general consumption, so to speak—that it was a particularly monastic practice, something best suited for monks and nuns living in seclusion. When we put this question to the monastics we met, we were half-expecting that they would reassure us with a breezy reply that this form of prayer is possible for anyone. To our surprise, when we asked this question, most of the monks and nuns were guarded in their answers. Under gentle but persistent inquiry, the reason for their reluctance to recommend the Jesus Prayer to everyone became clear: they could not imagine how someone with a family, a career, and bills to pay could sustain the level of intense mental focus that they took for granted as standard operating procedure when praying the Jesus Prayer.

The monks and nuns we spoke with echoed the point of view that had been expressed in spiritual texts of the last two millennia regarding the life of prayer in general, and the Jesus Prayer in particular: no one should begin such a program except under the supervision and direction of a wise, experienced spiritual guide. The monks and nuns weren't being proprietary; they were speaking from centuries of experience.

Living in the desert as an ascetic dedicated to prayer, whether in ancient times or today, means living in an extreme environment. Clearly an inexperienced person could hardly just walk out of ordinary life and into seclusion, into celibacy, and into extreme focus of the mind without the guidance of a spiritual director to help him or her make the transition. Individuals who have attempted the "go it alone" approach to the spiritual life have often gotten into trouble. There are many recorded instances of hermits hallucinating and suffering mental, physical, and emotional breakdowns because they had been careless of their health and diet in their excessively zealous dedication to prayer. We are talking of extremists who attempted to live solely on bread and water, who routinely devoted the entire night to prayer and permitted themselves only an hour of sleep at a time. In their zeal for the things of the Spirit, these ascetics ruined their physical and mental health—tragically, without making any progress toward their sacred goal.

Men such as St. Basil (c. 330–379) in the East and St. Benedict (c. 480–550) in the West embraced the idea of renunciation of life's luxuries, but they moderated the penances that earlier practitioners had imposed upon themselves. In the rules Basil and Benedict composed for their monks, they recognized the value of the old penitential forms and made them part of monastic life—but in a modified form. As Benedicta Ward, a historian of the religious life, tells us, "The monks went without sleep because they were watching for the Lord; they did not speak because they were listening to God; they fasted because they were fed by the Word of God. It was the end that mattered, the ascetic practices were only a means."

It is important to understand that praying the Jesus Prayer by no means requires assuming the life of a cloistered monk. It is not necessary to go without sleep, or begin fasts or penances, in order to integrate prayer into one's life. Some of the monks and nuns we spoke with cautioned that suddenly attempting to pray constantly or assume ascetic practices outside a monastery might even be detrimental, and should be avoided. When people enter the monastic life, they begin as complete novices guided by mentors, spending years working up to the practice of constant prayer. It's not something to jump into suddenly, or without guidance.

Nonetheless, we came away from our conversations with an overall sense that the Jesus Prayer can be a useful tool for anyone seeking a deeper spiritual life. Yes, the richest rewards may come in a life dedicated to prayer and contemplation, but what makes the Jesus Prayer so extraordinary is that its abundant graces are not limited to the monastic life. It can enrich the life of anyone who prays it faithfully and with concentration. The point is to add prayer into your existing routine, not to change your lifestyle in order to become a monk, or monklike.

In fact, our friend His Eminence Metropolitan Daniel Ciobotea of Iaşi in Romania observed that the breakdown of community life in urban and suburban areas may actually be conducive to developing a richer life of prayer. "Today some great cities, big cities—*megalopolises*—are similar to the desert," he said. "Although there are crowds of people, many persons are feeling like [they are] in the desert because there is not enough communion, not enough communication, and I think the [Jesus] Prayer is to transform the solitude into communion, and first of all communion with God, fellowship with God."

An Entire Theology

Two of the most important facets of praying the Jesus Prayer are contemplation and stillness. The purpose of Christian contemplation is to experience God directly, to put oneself in the presence or awareness of the Divine. There are many forms of contemplation in many religions, but contemplation in Christianity is significantly different, because the Presence that Christians seek in contemplation is not an abstraction or a beautiful idea but the incarnate Jesus Christ, God the Son, the Second Person of the Holy Trinity, who as the Bible says came down from heaven and for the salvation of the world became man.

In mystical texts stillness (or silence) often goes by its Greek name, *hesychia*. It is a form of prayer and meditation, but also a heightened

The Secrets of the Bridal Chamber

Throughout our pilgrimage Father John and I met monks and nuns who hinted at the inexpressible spiritual joys they experienced when they came into the presence of God. When we asked them for more details, they demurred, but none more tellingly than Mother Maria, a sister at the Agapia Monastery in Romania. "It's not possible," she said, "to openly discuss the delights of the blessedness of the meeting between the bride and the Bridegroom." The bride is Mother Maria's metaphor for the soul, and the Bridegroom is Jesus Christ.

Here, then, are a few reflections on the intense spiritual joys that some of the holy men and women we encountered have experienced in the Jesus Prayer:

A child keeps quiet when she feels the arms of her parents and feels the joy of being with her parents. And I think it is the same feeling when a novice comes and when she finds silence. When she finds herself in such an environment she feels the love of God, and she feels that joy which that little child would in the parents' arms.

SISTER JOSEPHINA,

ABBESS OF VĂRATEC MONASTERY, ROMANIA

consciousness in which one is immersed in the grace of God. Those who have experienced it say that it is intangible and indescribable.

As for the Jesus Prayer, it contains a whole theology within itself, to paraphrase Father Lazarus, a monk of St. Antony's Monastery in Egypt. Here's the message that father Lazarus hears in the various parts of "Lord Jesus Christ, Son of God, have mercy on me, a sinner":

Lord is the title that establishes the authority or dominion of Jesus Christ.

God is love, God is quietness, God is peace; and if I feel love and peace in my heart, I know that I am close to God.

SISTER ANGELINA,

POKROVSKY MONASTERY, KIEV, UKRAINE

When we pray, we are actually similar to the angels who are in a state of ceaseless praise for God.

FATHER SERAFIM,

MONASTERY OF ST. ANA, ROHIA, ROMANIA

We cannot talk about asceticism if we don't have humility. We are talking now about mental prayer. If there is no humility, it's just lip service. If we have humility, then the prayer comes into the heart and we feel warmth in the heart, which causes the heart to rejoice. And this joy of the heart is a sign of the action of the Holy Spirit.

HIS EMINENCE ARCHBISHOP DAMIANOS,

MONASTERY OF ST. CATHERINE, MOUNT SINAI

Without prayer a monk is just a man in a black dress.

FATHER JONAS,

MONASTERY OF ST. JONAS, KIEV, UKRAINE

Jesus is the Latin form of his Aramaic and Hebrew name, *Yeshua,* which means "salvation." It is related to another Hebrew name, *Yahoshua* (Joshua in English), which means "Lord who is salvation."

Christ comes from the Greek word *Christos,* which means "the anointed one." The Hebrew form of this word is *Messias* (Messiah in English).

Son of God is meant literally. Jesus is the Second Person of the Holy Trinity, begotten by God the Father. For the salvation of the world he came down from heaven and was born of the Blessed Virgin Mary. He is the Son of God and the son of Mary, fully God and fully human. As is always the case when trying to explain the doctrine of the Trinity, we are in an area of absolute sacred mystery, which no mind can comprehend.

Have mercy on me, a sinner. The Greek for "Lord, have mercy," *Kyrie eleison,* is one of the oldest prayers of the Christian liturgy. It is derived from the parable of the Pharisee and the tax collector in St. Luke's Gospel (18:10–14). Two men enter the Temple in Jerusalem. The Pharisee goes up to the front, where he thanks God "that I am not like other men" (v. 11). Then the Pharisee lists all the splendid things he does, as if he were trying to impress God. As for the tax collector, he stands at the back of the Temple and will not even raise his eyes; instead, he strikes his breast with his fist as he prays, "God, be merciful to me, a sinner!" (v. 13). This final phrase of the Jesus Prayer is an admission of personal failings, of error, of spiritual sickness; it is an act of repentance; and it is a petition that begs for God's mercy and forgiveness. It is also a prayer that finds special favor with God, for as Jesus explained to his disciples after telling them this parable, "I tell you, this man [the tax collector] went down to his house justified rather than the other; for all who exalts will be humbled, but every one who humbles himself will be exalted" (v. 14).

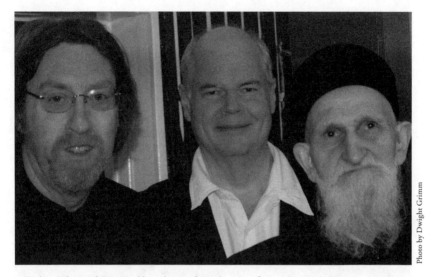

Father John and Norris Chumley with Father Serafim at St. Ana's Monastery, near Rohia, Romania. *Serafim* means "angel," and this monk truly fits that description.

Many people practice the Jesus Prayer for half an hour or fifteen minutes at a time, and for them it can be a revelatory experience. For those who practice it for long hours at a stretch over days and days, it is a different matter. Then it can literally restructure deep patterns of thinking, dislocating people from ordinary life so that they can commune with God. It was not by accident, of course, that the great practitioners of the Jesus Prayer could not sustain ordinary lives (by which I mean predominantly lives in a city environment, with bodies and minds that needed to get themselves to work in the morning and had to juggle the numerous demands of family, friends, co-workers, clients, and supervisors).

So for what follows, let me make it clear that I am not writing for people thinking of adopting the ascetical practice of uninterrupted prayer. I am thinking only of the many who are looking for a practice of prayer that can help them focus their attention, deepen their perception of spiritual things, and calm the innumerable distractions that so often deflect us from spiritual attentiveness and peace.

Let us begin.

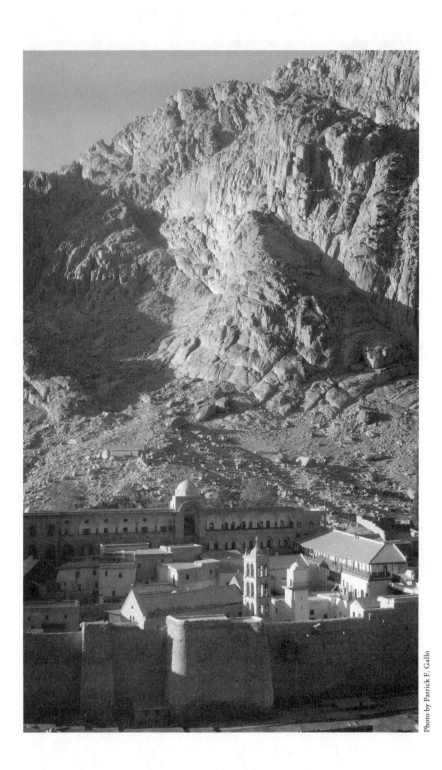

2

The Living Tradition of the Jesus Prayer

The Monasteries of St. Antony and St. Catherine

F ATHER JOHN AND I, along with his wife and our film crew, crossed the Egyptian desert in a modern van and could hardly complain about a lack of comfort. Nonetheless, the journey was difficult: driving hundreds of miles through a hot, barren, featureless landscape left us emotionally and psychologically exhausted. The harsh, unforgiving glare of the sun blasted through the van's windows, forcing us to squint and avert our eyes.

We were on our way to the Monastery of St. Antony, the oldest Christian monastery in the world, in quest of that spiritual, interior peace which the ancient Christians had known but which most

---

Opposite: St. Catherine's Monastery at the foot of Mount Sinai, Egypt, taken from Mount Horeb. Note the wooden entryway near the top of the front wall; this is the original monastery entrance. Visitors had to be hoisted up by rope, riding in a basket. Of the two near towers, the one on the left (with the arches) is the bell tower of the ancient church; the one on the right tops a chapel built for visiting Muslims.

contemporary Christians have lost. Yet everywhere we traveled in Egypt we were accompanied by an armed guard. Every time I spoke with him I could see it peeping out from beneath his jacket. To our readers it may seem incongruous, but it was a necessity; in recent years Egypt has seen too many outbreaks of violence against Egyptian Christians and foreign tourists. I appreciated that our hosts were taking no chances with us.

Egypt is unique in the history of Christianity: it is the only place outside Israel where Jesus lived. The second chapter of St. Matthew's Gospel tells us that when King Herod tried to murder the Christ Child, the Virgin Mary and St. Joseph fled with him into Egypt. It is assumed that the Holy Family found sanctuary among Egypt's Jewish community, which was sizable in the first century AD. The Coptic Orthodox Church, the largest Christian denomination in Egypt, has created the Holy Family Trail, which identifies more than a dozen locations traditionally associated with Jesus, Mary, and Joseph, including a cave beneath the Greek cemetery in Cairo said to be where the Holy Family hid from Herod's soldiers, and the Church of St. Mark in Assiut, built over the spot where it is believed an angel appeared to St. Joseph bearing the message that Herod was dead and it was safe to return to Israel.

According to a venerable tradition, the evangelist St. Mark carried the gospel to Egypt about the year AD 45 and remained in the country to serve as the first bishop of Alexandria. One of the oldest Christian catechetical schools in the world was opened in 190 in Alexandria; it was the training ground for such great theologians as St. Clement of Alexandria (c. 150–c. 217) and Origen (c. 185–254), and it attracted theologians and biblical scholars from throughout the Mediterranean world, including the great St. Jerome (c. 341–420), who produced the first authoritative Latin translation of the Bible.

Egyptian Christians take pride in their title, "the Church of the Martyrs." They believe that their long history of martyrdom began on the day after Easter, May 8, AD 68, when Roman soldiers seized St. Mark and dragged him by his heels through the streets of Alexandria until he was dead. In the anti-Christian persecutions that flared up time and again over the next three centuries, Egyptian Christians such as St. Apollonia (died c. 249), St. Maurice and his companions in the Theban Legion (died c. 287), St. Menas (died c. 300), and St. Catherine of Alexandria (died c. 306), along with countless others—men, women, and even children—gave their lives rather than betray their faith. Since 641, when Egypt was conquered by the armies of Islam, Christians in the country have suffered periods of persecution, sometimes government-sponsored, sometimes the result of anti-Christian mass hysteria. Riots broke out a few years back, for example, when a rumor spread that Christians were sprinkling a magic liquid on Muslim women's burkas that caused little crosses to materialize on the fabric.

As much as Father John and I admire and venerate the martyrs of Egypt, we had come to experience a different facet of Egypt's spiritual life. Egypt is the cradle of monasticism, beginning with St. Paul the Hermit and St. Antony of the Desert, whom we introduced in the previous chapter. That's why Father John and I had gone to Egypt: to immerse ourselves in a form of monastic life that has scarcely changed in 1,700 years, and to discover the wisdom of both ancient and contemporary practitioners of the Jesus Prayer.

"It's a Short Walk"

From a distance across the desert we could see two tall, thin towers, each crowned with a large gold-colored cross. This was the gate of St. Antony's Monastery, the oldest continuously inhabited monastery in the Christian world, founded in 356, the year the saint died. It lies at the base of Al-Qalzam Mountain near Al-Zaafarana, not very far from the Red Sea—truly out in the middle of nowhere, which is exactly what St. Antony had in mind. As is true with all ascetics, he believed that the monastic life could be lived authentically only in places remote from large population centers. "The wax melts when it comes near the fire," said St. Antony, "and thus the virtues of the ascetic disappear when he is in proximity with the world." In a cliff 680 meters above the Red Sea and about two kilometers from the monastery is the cave where St. Antony lived for the last forty-six years of his life.

Like most monasteries, St. Antony's is largely a self-sufficient community, a miniature village with a mill, a bakery, vegetable gardens, and accommodations for guests. It also preserves in its library a remarkable collection of 1,700 rare manuscripts. The library once contained many more, but years ago the monastery's Bedouin servants tragically used some of the dry parchments to start cooking fires. There are also five churches within the monastery walls, dating from the seventh through the thirteenth centuries, all of them adorned with murals. The murals have all been cleaned recently: Egypt's Supreme Council of Antiquities, working in collaboration with the American Research Center in Egypt, brought in a team of specialists to remove centuries of candle soot, dust, and grime, revealing the paintings' original brilliant colors.

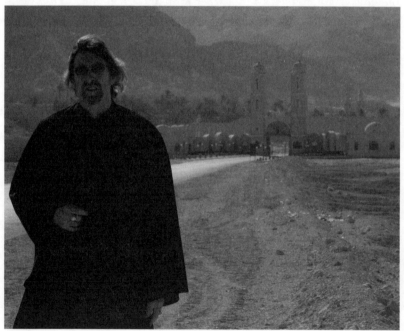

Photo by Norris J. Chumley

Father John McGuckin on the road to St. Antony's Monastery,
near the Egyptian Red Sea.

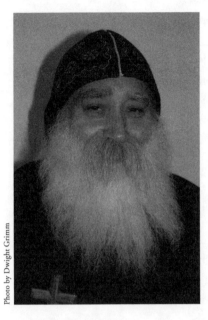

Photo by Dwight Grimm

Father Ruwais, the English-speaking guide and father at St. Antony's Monastery.

Today the monastery is home to approximately 150 monks, and welcomes pilgrims who come to pray inside St. Antony's cave. We arrived at the monastery just as an elderly monk with a very long white beard and wearing an unusual black cap embroidered with small white crosses was about lead a group of visitors around the monastery. The monk introduced himself to us as Father Ruwais, gave us permission to film in the monastery, and promised to give us an interview later. But first he had a tour to conduct, so Father John and I tagged along. We already had obtained permission and invitations in advance, including a blessing from the archbishop of the Coptic Church, but no one on the monastery grounds was aware of that groundwork. This, we would soon discover, would become a pattern.

Father Ruwais was a natural guide, a born showman, who pointed out to us the monastery's most interesting treasures and took us to drink from a spring near one of the churches. "This is where Moses struck water in the desert," he said, "and the spring still flows today." Next he served us refreshments: freshly baked pita bread, carried in on a large wooden board by a boy named (appropriately) Moses. Finally, he herded us into the gift shop, which actually had many wonderful and inexpensive items.

I was eager to interview Father Ruwais, but he put us off. "I am tired and must rest. I recently had heart surgery and must take a nap for an hour. It is just enough time for you and your colleagues to climb up the steps to visit St. Antony's cave! Go, it's just behind the monastery. You will find your way. I will meet you back here in one hour. It's a short walk."

"He Is Still Here"

The mountain behind the monastery is incredibly beautiful, offering vistas that seem to stretch for hundreds of miles. Once we got beyond the monastery walls we could see no one, and we heard no sounds except spirited winds. As for the short walk Father Ruwais had mentioned, it was in fact a long climb—over 1,100 steps, cut into the living rock of the mountain—that led up to St. Antony's cave.

At the top of the staircase, jutting into the mountain from a craggy ledge, was a cave about five feet tall and two feet wide. From 310 until 356 this had been St. Antony's home. There were a couple of teenaged Muslim boys there, paying homage to the hermit, but aside from our little group there was no one else. The interior was narrow, cramped, and dark, but we had a headlamp and a flashlight with us. With these we examined the little altar upon which stood icons of Christ and St. Antony, as well as a bunch of dried flowers. Behind the altar we found a crevice where St. Antony must have curled up and slept all those years.

St. Antony's cave is one of the holiest places I've ever been. The total peace that I felt, so far away from everything and everyone, was very moving. In the stillness of the cave Father John and his wife, Eileen, began to sing Christian chants.

In this extraordinary place we lost track of time. Three hours had passed unnoticed, and we had promised to meet Father Ruwais two hours earlier! We raced down the stairs and back to the monastery. The gates were shut, but the monk at the entryway recognized us, let us in, and called Father Ruwais—on a walkie-talkie.

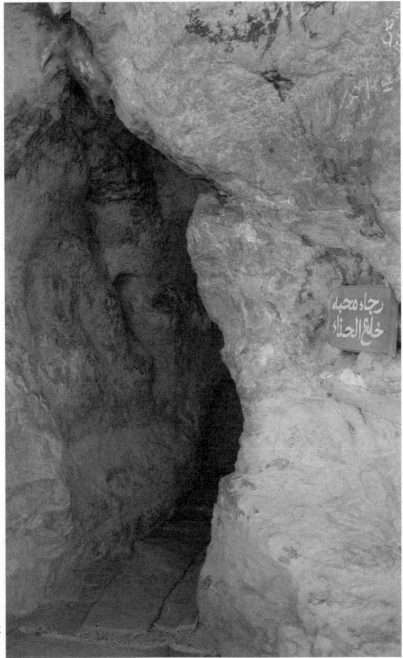

Photo by John A. McGuckin

The entrance to St. Antony's cave at the top of Al-Qalzam Mountain.
Note the graffiti, some of which is centuries old.

A few moments later Father Ruwais arrived and led Father John and me into a chapel where the monks were chanting vespers. As we listened, Father Ruwais whispered to me, "You're the first to ever film us about the content of the prayers, and what's in our heart." At the conclusion of vespers, the abbot rose from his place and greeted us, followed by a smallish monk who appeared from a distant corner, took me by the arm, and led me outside the chapel.

"God told me you were coming," he said. "You're making a very important contribution to the world. Come with me up the mountain to my cave, and we can talk on-camera." I was taken aback. Who was this? Seeing my confusion, he said, "I'm Father Lazarus, the starets of the community." That meant I was talking to the spiritual master of the monastery, and he had invited us to film him, a living hermit, inside his own cave. God is an amazing producer.

It was nearly sundown, which made filming in Father Lazarus's cave impossible, but he was imperturbable. He suggested an alternate site—inside the main church, at the tomb of St. Antony. Father Ruwais agreed to come, too.

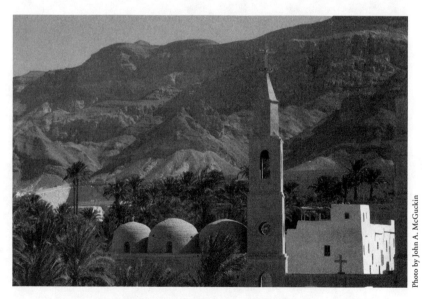

St. Antony Church at St. Antony's Monastery.

Photo by John A. McGuckin

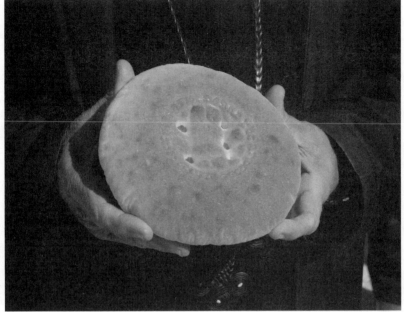

Photo by John A. McGuckin

Holy bread for Eucharist, St. Antony's Monastery.

Father Lazarus had been at St. Antony's for thirty years, he told us. Before that he had been an atheist, a professor of Marxist philosophy and economics in his native New Zealand. One day he felt a powerful and unexpected call to convert to Christianity and to travel to Egypt to seek God at St. Antony's Monastery. He has been there ever since.

Sitting beside the resting place of St. Antony, in a chapel lit by candles, Father Lazarus spoke to us of his vocation: "I wanted to come to the desert to offer [God] whatever love I could give him through prayer and to receive from God, one to one, this kind of spiritual knowledge. And I found it here—in St. Antony's desert life, in this mountain, I have found it. So that's why [I chose] the solitary life in the desert, particularly in this desert where St. Antony was the father who started this special Christian life, this monastic life. To sit here at his feet and feel his power—because he is still here, he is not departed, and he remains our father, our living father—so to be here with him helps me to feel the love of God through prayer."

Guns in the Desert

After St. Antony's Monastery, our next stop was the Monastery of St. Catherine on Mount Sinai, a place renowned throughout the Christian world, yet incredibly difficult to get to. There's this big hurdle to go over—or rather, around—called the Red Sea. You can drive from Cairo to Mount Sinai, but it takes many hours; the only road is narrow and dangerous, and you cannot go quickly. But from Cairo you can catch a plane to Sharm al-Sheikh, a resort town at the foot of the Red Sea; from there it is only a four-hour drive to Mount Sinai.

The Wisdom of Father Lazarus of St. Antony's Monastery

Father Lazarus offered us his thoughts on prayer, silence, and the value of spiritual struggles:

On Prayer

Prayer is two-way. You have to say, you have to *speak* your prayer, but you also have to listen. You see, if you're not listening, how is God going to answer you?

On Silence

First of all, there are kinds of silence. There is silence and there is silence. Silence can mean not speaking; you are going to stay in a place that is quiet. This is helpful. It's nice to go into a nice forest or a nice garden where you are away from traffic and from talking with people, where you are away from the demands of the modern world. But this is an exterior silence—which helps you breathe slowly, to enjoy the aesthetic pleasure, the beauty of the creation—but it is transient; it will not last.

The drive to Mount Sinai took us through a landscape of rocks upon rocks, intermingled in places with sand. In this apparently God-forsaken place, God made himself known to Moses, and then to the Israelites, and then to the hermits and monks who have dwelt here since at least the fourth century. The monks refer to Sinai as "God-trodden," and to my mind it truly is a God-trodden place, where for thousands of years people have come to escape the throes and woes of civilization while waiting for God to appear.

About every ten miles across the Sinai desert there is a checkpoint: a road barricade and one-story tower with a gunman pointing his

There is another type of silence which is interior silence. Now this is much harder to find, but it is long-lasting. For example, memories. Here we are living in the desert; here I am living up there in the mountain. For long periods of time—two weeks, three weeks, one month—I don't see any people. I'm not committing sins of action daily. I'm just sitting quietly and working and praying and being alone. What about my mind? My mind can range everywhere. If I don't have interior silence, I can be as busy in mind as if I were in New York.

On Spiritual Struggles

Most of my life is struggle. I must fight against temptations; I must fight against weakness. So I actually think that the truest spiritual life is not permanent peace with calm and no worries. This can be a state of delusion. The truest spiritual life, the best spiritual life, is one when there are these moments of peace. The Lord grants them because he loves us.

But a lot of the time we struggle, we fight. By this we show the Lord that we are on the way to him; we are doing something for him, even as he struggled for us.

automatic rifle out the window. Some of the guards were working for the Egyptian government, others were Camp David Accord United Nations peacekeepers, and still others were members of some type of militia. They were all heavily armed and scary-looking. Nonetheless, we did not have any trouble; after our guide for this part of the journey, Akmed, explained who we were and why we were there, the checkpoint guards let us proceed.

Given the region's volatile, unpredictable recent history, Egypt can be a foreboding place. I knew we were not far from Israel, Palestine, and the Gaza Strip. Not far from Syria. Not far from Somalia, and Sudan, and Darfur. I was grateful that Akmed had had the foresight to bring along a guard, the young man I mentioned earlier; dressed in a suit and tie, he carried a semiautomatic pistol and walked with us every step we took.

A Mystical Marriage

Mount Sinai is sacred to Jews, Christians, and Muslims; it is the place where God spoke to Moses from out of the burning bush and where he gave Moses the Ten Commandments. The empress mother of Constantine, St. Helena (c. 250–330), made a pilgrimage to the Holy Land from 325 to 327. During her visit she ordered a chapel constructed on Sinai, at the spot where the burning bush was then believed to have stood. That chapel, known today as St. Helena's, survives within the walls of St. Catherine's Monastery, as does a flourishing bush said to be the one from which God spoke. For Father John and me, Mount Sinai has additional significance: some say the practice of the Jesus Prayer began here.

By the end of the fourth century, hermits and monks had gathered around this sacred site, but they were frequent targets of Bedouin raiders. To protect the holy men, Emperor Justinian I (483–565) had a walled monastery built here, a project that took nearly forty years to complete. Justinian's monastery, which has never been destroyed, preserves an astonishing collection of ancient icons and manuscripts, including the Codex Sinaiticus. Dating from about 350, that Greek manuscript is one of the oldest surviving copies of the Bible. The monastery library also preserves certified copies of a letter from the Prophet Muhammad guaranteeing the safety of the monks and their monastery; the original was taken to Constantinople in 1517 by the command of Sultan Selim I, who confirmed the privileges Muhammad had promised and sent the copies to the monks as a pledge that he and his successors would honor the word of the Prophet.

Toward the end of the first millennium AD, the monks of Sinai discovered the remains of the martyr St. Catherine of Alexandria. According to legend, she was a young woman of great intelligence who had studied Greek and Roman philosophy and was a frequent visitor to the great library of Alexandria. One day, as she was reading in the library, she fell asleep and dreamed of a beautiful woman with a delightful little boy sitting in her lap. Pointing to Catherine, the mother said to the child, "Would you like to marry her?" The little boy replied, "Oh no! She is so ugly!" At that, Catherine woke up, weeping.

Nearby was an elderly gentleman who approached and asked if he could be of assistance. Catherine said she was crying because of a dream she'd just had. The stranger asked her to tell him her dream, and when she had, he said, "I am a Christian priest, and I can tell you what your dream meant. The lady was the Blessed Virgin Mary, and the little boy was Jesus Christ, her Son. He found you ugly because, although you possess wisdom, you are still a pagan and your unbaptized soul is stained with many sins."

"How can I make myself beautiful for him?" Catherine asked the priest.

"I will instruct you in the Christian faith and baptize you," the priest said, "and then Christ the Lord will delight in the beauty of your soul."

Catherine took his instruction and was baptized. Once again she dreamed of Mary and Jesus. This time, when Mary asked if Jesus would like to marry Catherine, he said, "Oh yes! Because now she is truly beautiful." With that, he placed a ring on Catherine's finger; and when she woke up, the ring was on her hand. This incident, known as the Mystical Marriage of St. Catherine, was a popular subject with artists of the Renaissance and Baroque eras—painters such as Veronese, Rubens, van Dyck, and Correggio.

During Emperor Diocletian's empire-wide persecution of Christians in the early fourth century, Catherine was arrested and ordered to offer sacrifice to the Roman gods. She refused. Moved by her beauty and intelligence, the judge brought in fifty pagan philosophers to convince Catherine that her faith was misplaced. Instead of being persuaded to renounce Christianity, Catherine converted the philosophers. She was sentenced to be torn to pieces on a spiked wheel, but the moment she touched it, the wheel shattered. Enraged, the judge ordered Catherine beheaded. After her death, angels carried her body to Mount Sinai and buried it in a secret place, where it remained undisturbed until 800, when the Sinai monks discovered the grave. They carried the martyr's relics back to their church, where they placed them in a marble sarcophagus. Today, the saint's relics are enshrined in a gold and silver casket.

Elder Pavlos, one of the monks of Mount Sinai, told us, "St. Catherine stole the glory of the Old Testament saints—Moses, Aaron, etc., even the [glory of the] ascetics who lived before her in this place. For the love of Christ she sacrificed everything, even her own life. She was an extremely gifted person in this life. She was not just a simple person like myself. She had wisdom, beauty, and wealth—the daughter of a king. And all this she considered rubbish compared to the love of Christ. The same holds true for the monk. . . . Thus St. Catherine provides the nicest example for the monastic."

Peace Profound and Absolute

We were near St. Catherine's when we stopped at an oasis; there we encountered a Bedouin family selling trinkets by the side of the road: among them, little carved stone pyramids, handmade leather purses stitched together with camel hair, small toy drums. Two little kids, a boy and a girl, went with us as we climbed up a mesa that was a resting place for John Moschos and Sophronius during their pilgrimage in the seventh century.

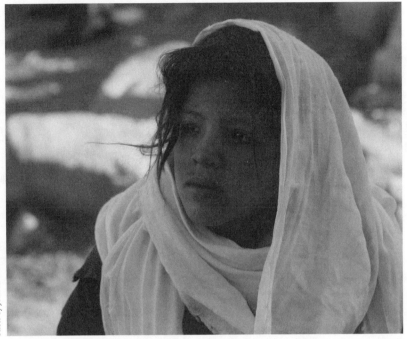

Photo by John A. McGuckin

Bedouin girl encountered on the way to St. Catherine's Monastery.

Three checkpoints later we arrived at last at the monastery's front gate. Nearby stood a visitors' center, swarming with tourists, and in that moment my impression of a peaceful, hidden sanctuary at the foot of Mount Sinai was shattered. There were tour buses everywhere, loading and unloading "pilgrims" who flocked to the souvenir shops to purchase St. Catherine's T-shirts and replicas of the monastery's most famous icons.

Thank God the monastery itself is protected from all that. Yes, tour buses come in, but the madding crowds are herded into corrals outside the sixth-century walls. For true pilgrims there are a dozen or so guest rooms that one can reserve for several nights, which is what we had done, so it was a bit disheartening to discover upon arrival that all the plans we had made in advance were of no use. No one at the monastery knew our names or expected us. The monk who had been my pre-visit contact at St. Catherine's, the one who had supposedly

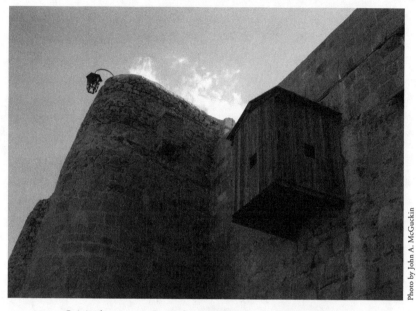

Photo by John A. McGuckin

Original entrance, St. Catherine's Monastery. Imagine having
to be hoisted up in a basket into the monastery through this doorway,
some fifty feet or so above the ground.

reserved our rooms and secured permission for us to film, was off in America supervising an installation of the monastery's magnificent icons at the J. Paul Getty Museum in Los Angeles.

We were asked to wait for Father Gregory, a monk who turned out to speak excellent English. With regret he informed us that the abbot was not aware of any advance plans, that none of the monks remembered hearing that we were coming. For a moment I feared that we were about to be turned away, but I succeeded in talking my way into the abbot's office, where I explained to the staff, as earnestly and sincerely as I could, the type of film we were making. Finally, after a few hours of anxious waiting, we were escorted into the private rooms of Archbishop Damianos, who was not only abbot of St. Catherine's but also the Archbishop of Sinai.

Father John and I explained the film and said that our aim was to bring the great graces of the Jesus Prayer to the world. This the abbot liked. He gave us permission to film inside the monastery. Jubilant,

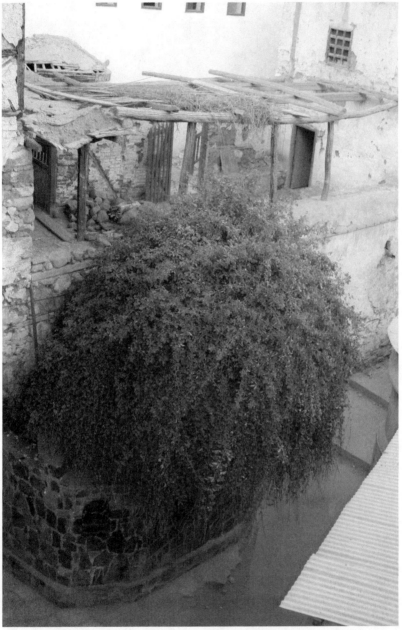

Photo by John A. McGuckin

In a corner of the courtyard of St. Catherine's Monastery behind a special masonry wall is the original burning bush—the one through which God spoke to Moses. The monks say that it has never stopped growing and thriving since the days of Moses. Its roots are under the chapel of the ancient church nearby.

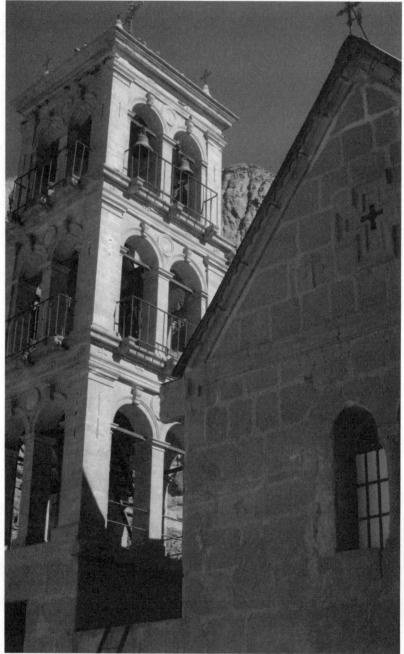

St. Catherine's Church of the Transfiguration and bell tower.

I kissed Archbishop Damianos's hand. Then he instructed Father Gregory to give us a grand tour, and to allow us to film anywhere and everywhere. I asked Father Gregory if we could include him in our film, but he declined. He was more than willing to act as our guide and interpreter in the monastery, he said, but humility would not permit him to appear on-camera.

St. Catherine's is a magical place. Nestled between Mount Sinai and Mount Horeb, the monastery is surrounded by solid stone walls approximately fifty feet high. Once the tourists were gone for the day, the peace inside those walls was profound and absolute.

We were up early the next morning for four hours of prayer in the church, which concluded with the Divine Liturgy. The sixth-century Church of the Transfiguration is a jewel. High above the altar, filling the arch of the sanctuary's half-dome, is one of the masterworks of Byzantine art, a sublime mosaic of the Transfiguration of Christ, flanked by Moses and Elijah, while the apostles—Sts. Peter, James, and John—cower before the vision in holy fear. The icons in the iconostasis, or altar screen (which separates the sanctuary from the main body of the church), as well as the icons that cover the walls and columns of the church are ancient, among the oldest in the world. The marble floor underfoot is uneven, worn by the feet of fifteen centuries of monks and pilgrims.

To our surprise, we were also invited to film inside the Holy of Holies (or inner sanctuary), the area around the altar, which is typically reserved for the clergy. It was an awe-inspiring experience to stand so close to the altar and film as the priest celebrated the Eucharist, the most solemn liturgy of the Orthodox Church.

Our peace and the solemnity of the place were shattered at 9:00 A.M. when the monks let the tourists in. There must be some who are quiet, sincere, devout, and respectful, but they get lost in the horde of rambunctious sightseers snapping flash photos nonstop as their tour guides talk loudly and incessantly. One of the monks told me that the tourists disturb his *hesychia,* his practice of prayer and stillness, and I certainly believe him.

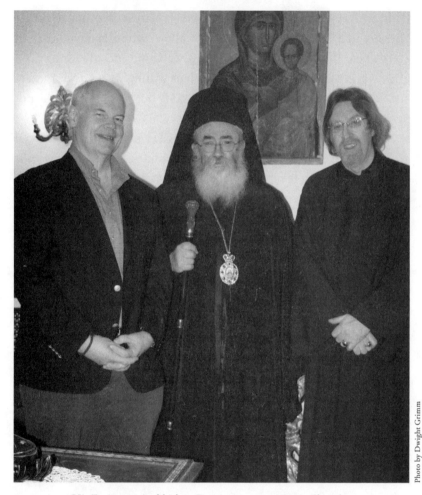

His Eminence Archbishop Damianos greets Norris Chumley
and Father John McGuckin at his offices in St. Catherine's Monastery.

Photo by Dwight Grimm

Archbishop Damianos is more sanguine, or perhaps charitable, about the visitors to St. Catherine's: "Naturally we have to occupy ourselves with hospitality, a *diakonima* [task] that we do while trying to decrease as much as possible the ensuing damage created to our *hesychia*. This is a *diakonima* of love to the visitors who come to this holy place for spiritual edification, to this place in which God himself walked, which is why it is called 'God-trodden Mount Sinai.' We, as monastics, are obligated on the one hand to serve these visitors and on the other hand to keep our *nous* [the seat of one's spiritual energy and the place where one becomes aware of the presence of God] focused on the [Jesus] Prayer. Not simply to say the prayer verbally, but with the heart. In the words of sacred Augustine, 'All our actions should be under the lens of eternity,' and by eternity we mean Christ."

The Alpha and the Omega

The monks allow the tourists to enter the monastery only between 9:00 A.M. and noon, Monday through Thursday and Saturday. In addition to being closed to visitors on Friday and Sunday, the monastery is closed on all the major feast days of the Greek Orthodox Church. It is not uncommon for visitors to arrive at St. Catherine's only to find the gates closed and locked because it is a holy day.

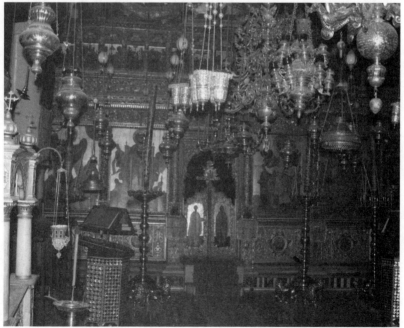

Photo by John A. McGuckin

Church of the Transfiguration, interior and iconostasis,
St. Catherine's Monastery.

The visitors are also restricted as to where they may go inside the monastery compound. They may visit the Chapel of the Burning Bush and the main church, the Basilica of the Holy Transfiguration, to see the works of art and to venerate, if they wish, relics of St. Catherine. Visitors must be completely silent inside the basilica, and as reminders the monks have posted signs that read, "This is a holy place; please treat it with respect."

I was surprised by the crowd of tourists and pilgrims that lined up behind a red velvet rope to venerate the relics. They stood silently as several monks covered a little table with red cloths, arranged candles and flowers on it, then removed from a gold-encrusted chest two reliquaries, one containing St. Catherine's skull, the other one of St. Catherine's hands. Once the velvet rope was lifted, the visitors surged forward, one at a time, to kiss the reliquaries. As a memento of the occasion, the monks gave each visitor a pot-metal ring stamped with an image of St. Catherine.

For nonbelievers the act of venerating the bones of a woman dead for 1,700 years may appear absurd. But for Orthodox and Catholic Christians it is not only a sign of love and respect, but also an act of humility in recognition of St. Catherine's steadfast faith. She experienced the action of the Holy Spirit within her soul, which gave her the courage to face a martyr's death. I expect many of the faithful who line up to venerate St. Catherine's relics hope to feel within their own hearts the warmth of holy joy the martyr knew.

As I was exiting the church, I heard a whispered, "Hello," aimed at me. There in a corner stood a monk robed in extra cassocks (it was cold that morning) looking right at me. I walked over to him. "Hi," I said, "I'm Norris."

"Father Neilos," he replied.

"You speak English!" I said. "There are not many here who do."

"Yes, I'm from England. We're very glad you're here. Nice to meet you." With that, he scurried away.

But we met again. Toward the end of our visit, as a special privilege, Father Neilos took us to see the ossuary. He led us to a little building and with a big set of keys unlocked multiple doors and gates until we entered a chamber piled high with bones: the earthly remains of thousands of Sinai monks. No tourist is ever admitted here.

The ossuary was unforgettable. The building may be only thirty feet by thirty feet, but it houses twenty or so display cases that preserve the bones of saints; one skeleton, St. Stephen, is dressed in a cassock and monk's cap. One section is reserved for the bones of abbots. Elsewhere the bones are arranged by type: skulls here, piled eight feet high; femurs and legs there; arms and hands elsewhere. "After a monk is buried for two or three years," Father Neilos explained, "we dig him up and save the bones. The skin has disappeared by then, unless it's a saint; then part of the skin remains, as [saints'] flesh is incorruptible."

I asked Father Neilos about the curious smell inside the ossuary. "Yes, indeed," he said, "the bones of monks give off myrrh, a sacred, fragrant oil that only the very high spiritual beings secrete." It truly was a unique fragrance, like musk oil mixed with citrus and herb. I had never smelled anything like it before. No cologne or perfume comes close. I thought of something Archbishop Damianos had said to me a few days earlier: "What is death? Death is the continuation of life without the body."

Before we left St. Catherine's I sat down with Father Neilos and asked him to talk about his life in the monastery and what part the Jesus Prayer plays in his spiritual life.

"Silence," Father Neilos said, "is really the most important thing. It's what unites the material with the immaterial. We know that the things of God cannot be learned; they are revealed. . . . I think God is always present and that's something that I'm always aware of. It's a bit like a prayer of words, but it is a silence. I think my relationship with God is in these words: 'Lord Jesus Christ, have mercy on me, a sinner.'"

"The Jesus Prayer," I said. "That says it all."

Father Neilos agreed. "That encompasses everything. Christ said he is Alpha and Omega—the prayer is that for me."

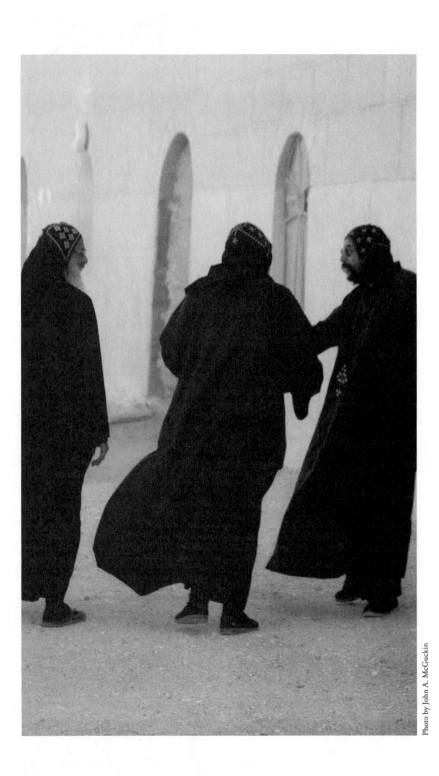

3

The Life-Transforming
Power of One Brief Prayer

THE EARLY CHRISTIANS were told, in 1 Thessalonians 5:16–18, to "rejoice always, pray without ceasing, give thanks in all circumstances; for this is the will of God in Christ for you." That has certainly always been the goal of the monastics.

The monks who went out into the desert centuries ago were expected by their spiritual masters to memorize all 150 songs in the book of Psalms. It is said that most if not all of those holy men could indeed recite each and every one by heart; some also memorized the four Gospels, and a select few are said to have memorized the entire Bible. The purpose of such ambitious memorization programs was to embed the words of sacred scripture in the consciousness of each monk, influencing how he spoke, how he thought, how he interpreted what he saw and experienced around him. Prayer, in other words, became his primary point of reference, the yardstick by which he measured all things.

The Divine Office, the prayers that monks and nuns of the churches in the East and in the West recite daily, draws heavily upon

Opposite: Monks at St. Antony's Monastery.

the book of Psalms. As for the Jesus Prayer, in the Eastern Church it is a private devotion; one could even say that for Eastern Christians it is the private prayer par excellence.

The Jesus Prayer is composed of two parts: it is a confession of faith—"Lord Jesus Christ, Son of God"—combined with an admission of sinfulness and a petition for help—"have mercy on me, a sinner." It recognizes Christ as the Son of God and the Savior of the world, who desires to reconcile all people to himself, and who possesses the power to forgive sins. In twelve words the Jesus Prayer summarizes the spiritual liberation proclaimed in the gospel and offers comfort and reassurance to whoever prays it. As such, the Jesus Prayer is a spiritual treasure of the Eastern Church, a treasure that could benefit many more if it became widely known in the West—which, of course, is the aim of this book.

Unlike other prayers, there is a method to reciting the Jesus Prayer that calls for controlling the body and focusing the mind. Orthodox

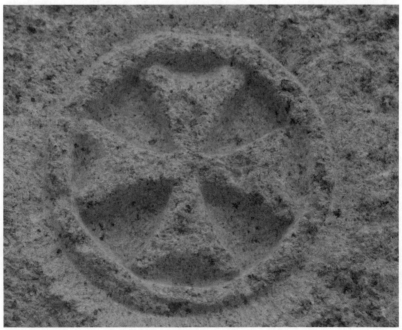

An ancient cross in the fortress wall, St. Catherine's Monastery.

Christians—clerics, religious, and laity—believe that when the practice of the Jesus Prayer is combined with receiving the sacraments, particularly the Eucharist, they can enter into a state of otherworldly peace where, free from all distractions, they enjoy a direct experience of God.

As a private prayer, the Jesus Prayer is not part of the liturgical life of the Orthodox Church; it is not even prayed aloud in a group as Catholics often pray the rosary, or as Protestants recite together the prayer of the day. It is profoundly personal: so much so that in Romania I met nuns who compared what they experienced while saying the Jesus Prayer to the secrets of a bridal chamber—something so sacred and intimate that it cannot be revealed.

Unbroken Union with God

The goal of one who begins to pray the Jesus Prayer is to fulfill St. Paul's injunction to the Christians of Thessalonica to pray without ceasing. St. Paul's instruction is echoed by St. John Climacus (c. 579–649) in his spiritual handbook, *The Ladder of Divine Ascent*. "Let the remembrance of Jesus be present with your every breath," St. John wrote. And he was not being metaphorical, for he was one of the champions of the constant recitation of the Jesus Prayer.

There is no complete biography of St. John Climacus, only a handful of details. He was born in Syria, or perhaps in what is now Israel, and was about sixteen years old when he entered the Monastery of St. Catherine on Mount Sinai. He remained there as a monk for several years, then asked to be released in order to live as a hermit in the Egyptian desert. At age seventy-five he was persuaded by the monks of St. Catherine to return to the monastery as their abbot. During the four years that he ruled the community he wrote *The Ladder of Divine Ascent*. (His surname, Climacus, comes from the Greek word for ladder.)

In his introduction to the *Philokalia*, Bishop Kallistos Ware of the Orthodox Church tells us that, after the Bible and the liturgical books of the Eastern Church, no work "has been studied, copied, and

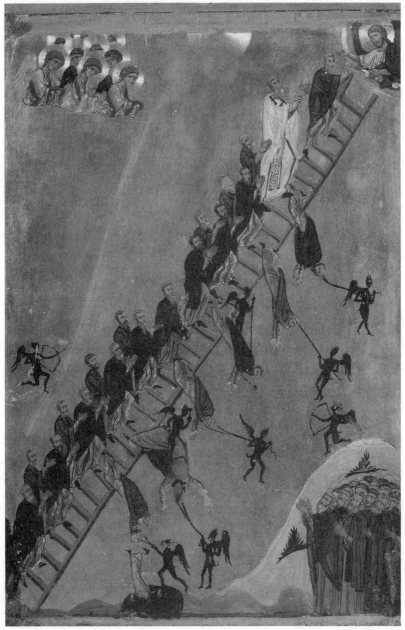

This icon, The Ladder of Divine Ascent, portrays the steps or rungs
on the ladder described by St. John Climacus in his book by the same title.
It is one of the world's oldest icons, now safely on display at St. Catherine's
Monastery, where St. John was once abbot.

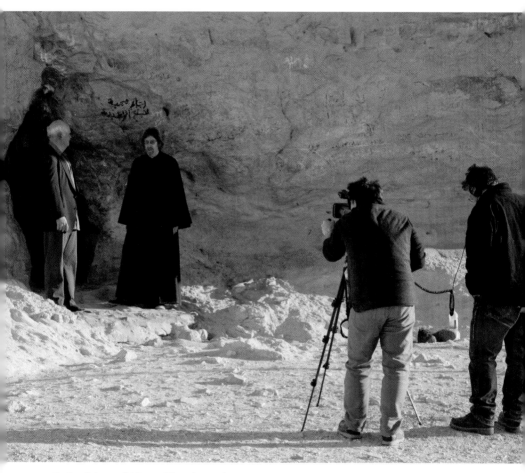

Father John and Norris Chumley at the entrance to St. Antony's cave, marveling at how he lived there for forty-six years, with only one loaf of bread and a jug of water a week, battling his demons. We are filmed by our directors of photography, Patrick Gallo and Dwight Grimm. (Photo by Ahmed Farid)

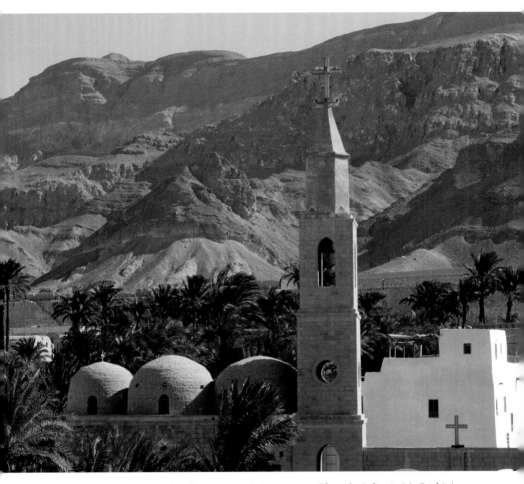

Above: St. Antony Church, St. Antony's Monastery. (Photo by John A. McGuckin)
Opposite: Refectory, St. Antony's Monastery. This is where the monks ate and heard prayers and parables for hundreds of years. Carved from stone, these are one-piece benches and a tabletop. They are no longer in use but are amazingly well preserved. (Photo by John A. McGuckin)

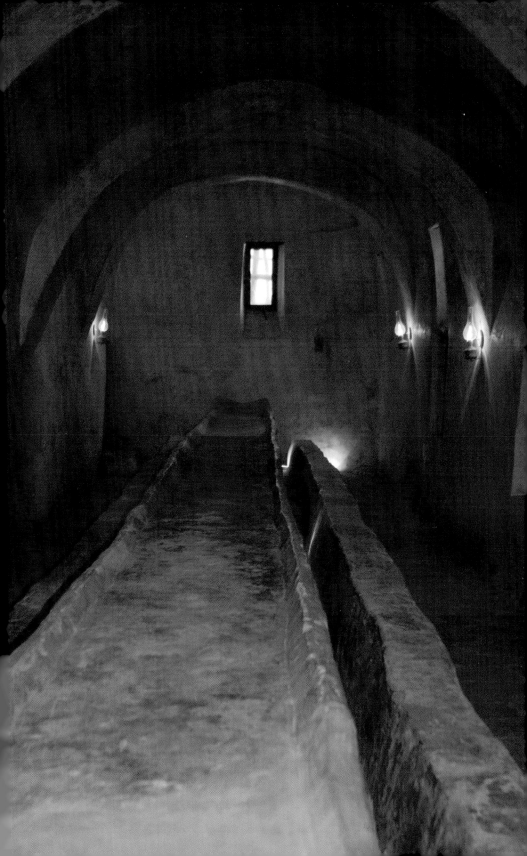

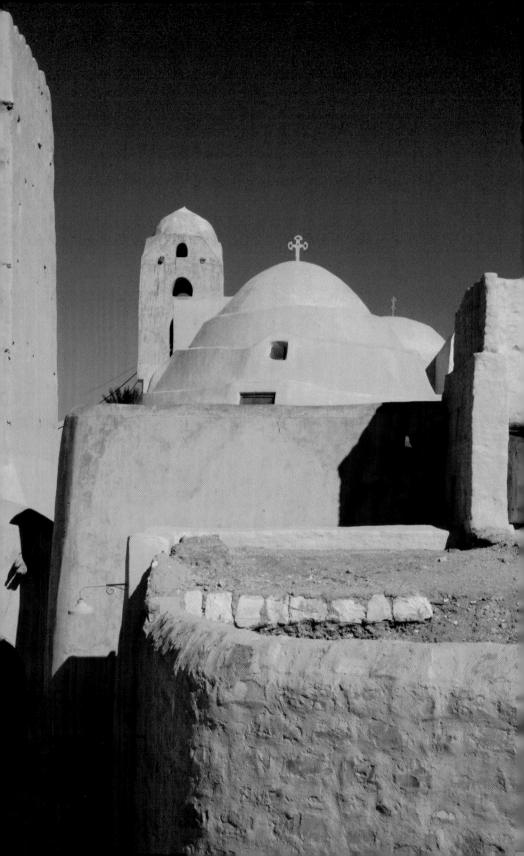

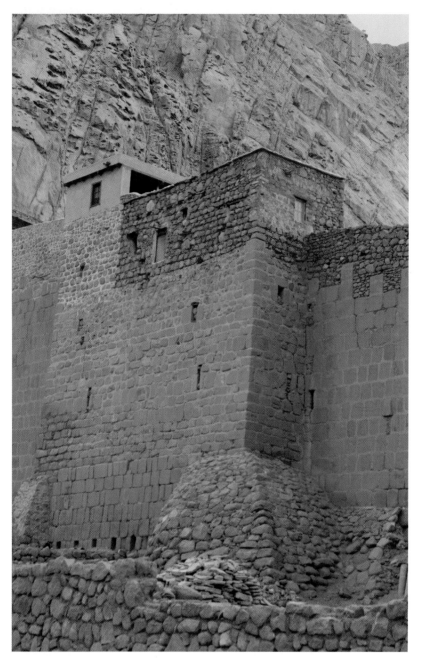

Opposite: Church exterior, St. Antony's Monastery. (Photo by John A. McGuckin)
Above: Late-fifth-century stone-walled fortress and fence at St. Catherine's Monastery, at the foot of Mount Sinai. (Photo by Norris J. Chumley)

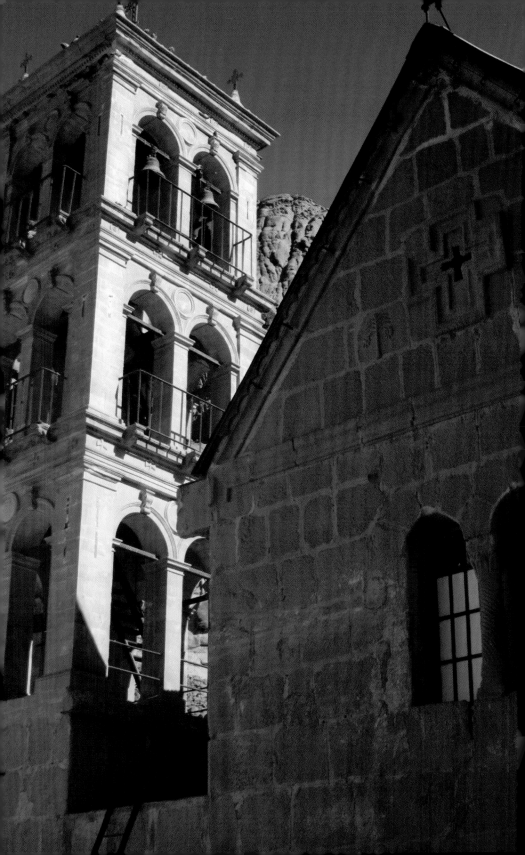

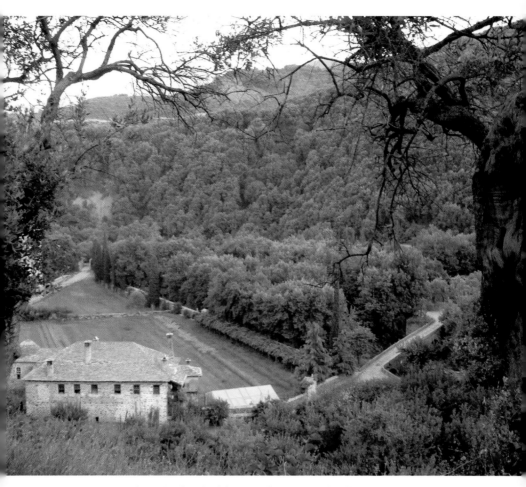

Opposite: St. Catherine's Church of the Transfiguration and bell tower.
(Photo by John A. McGuckin)
Above: A mystical grove of forest on the edge of Iviron Monastery, Mount Athos.
(Photo by Norris J. Chumley)

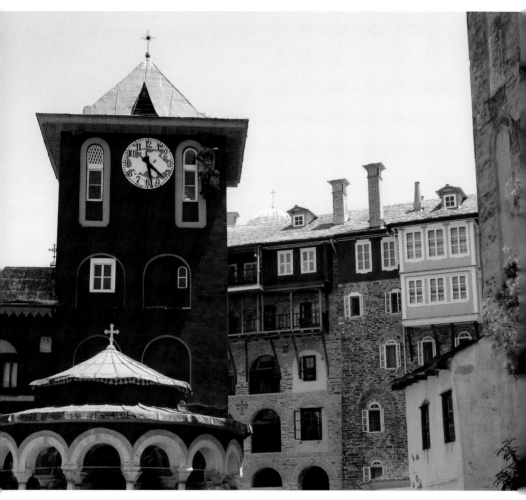

Vatopedi Monastery, Mount Athos. (Photo by Norris J. Chumley)

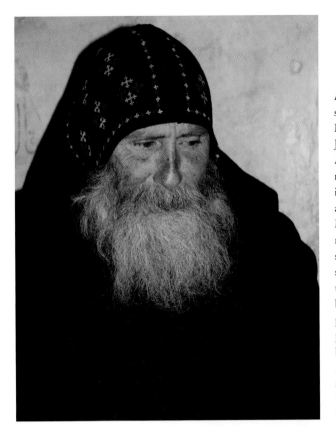

Left: Father Lazarus, starets of St. Antony's Monastery. (Photo by John A. McGuckin) *Below:* Father Jacob recites the Jesus Prayer in the bell tower high above Sergiyev Posad Monastery. It's a moment of peaceful solitude and seclusion floating above thousands of monks, bishops, archbishops, parishioners, and the patriarch gathered below. Hundreds of miles of Russian lands are visible behind him in the distance. (Photo by Dwight Grimm)

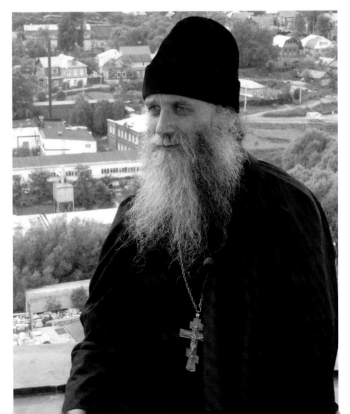

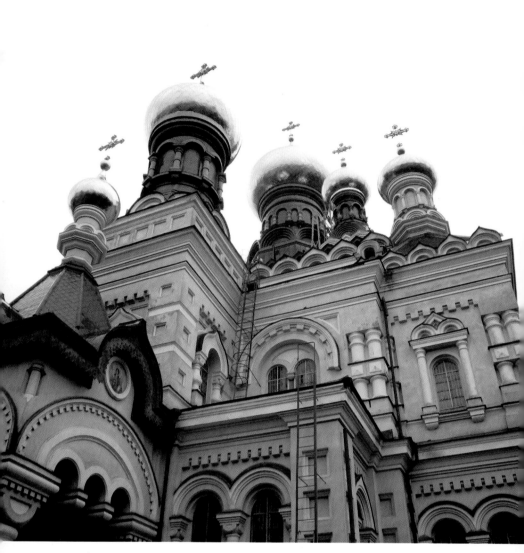

Above: Cathedral of St. Nicholas, Pokrovsky Monastery. (Photo by Dwight Grimm)
Opposite: Icon of the Mother of the Protective Veil, Pokrovsky Monastery. This is
an important and powerful image in Russia and Ukraine, with many churches and
monasteries dedicated to her. (Photo by Dwight Grimm)

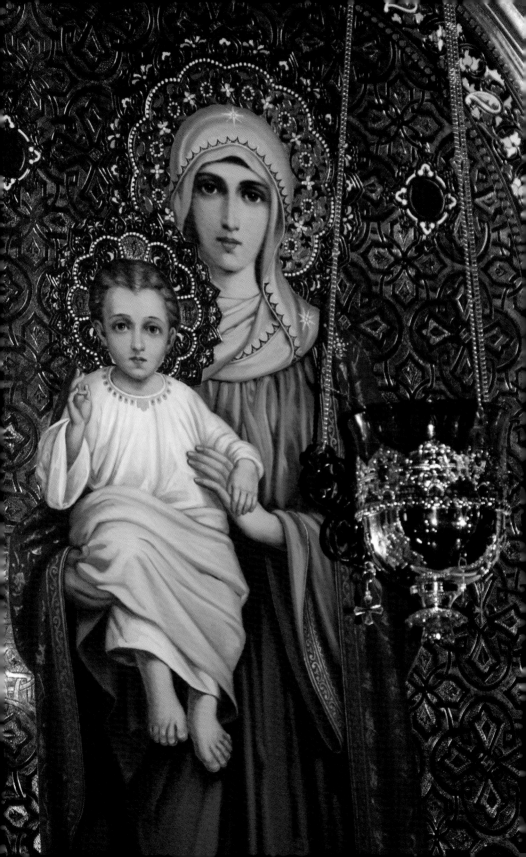

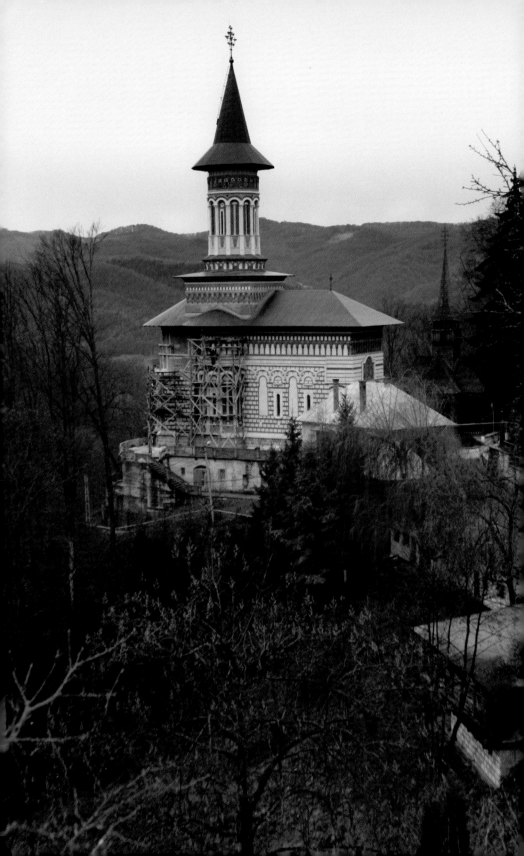

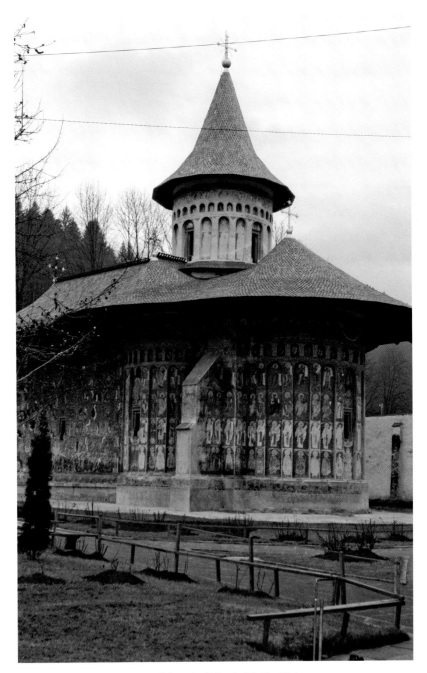

Opposite: St. Ana's Monastery. (Photo by John A. McGuckin)
Above: Voroneț Monastery church. Sometimes called the "Sistine Chapel of the East," the monastery has a fresco depicting the scenes of the Last Judgment, painted in 1547. Note the striking deep cerulean pigment of the scenes; it's called Voroneț Blue. (Photo by Norris J. Chumley)

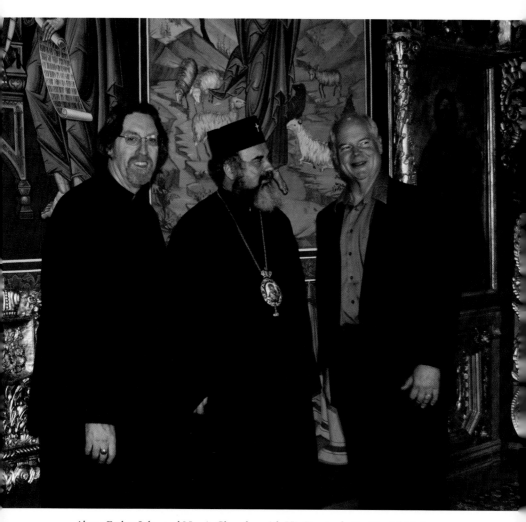

Above: Father John and Norris Chumley with His Beatitude Dr. Daniel Ciobotea, now patriarch of Romania. (Photo by Dwight Grimm) *Opposite:* The domes of Assumption Cathedral at Sergiyev Posad Monastery. (Photo by Dwight Grimm)

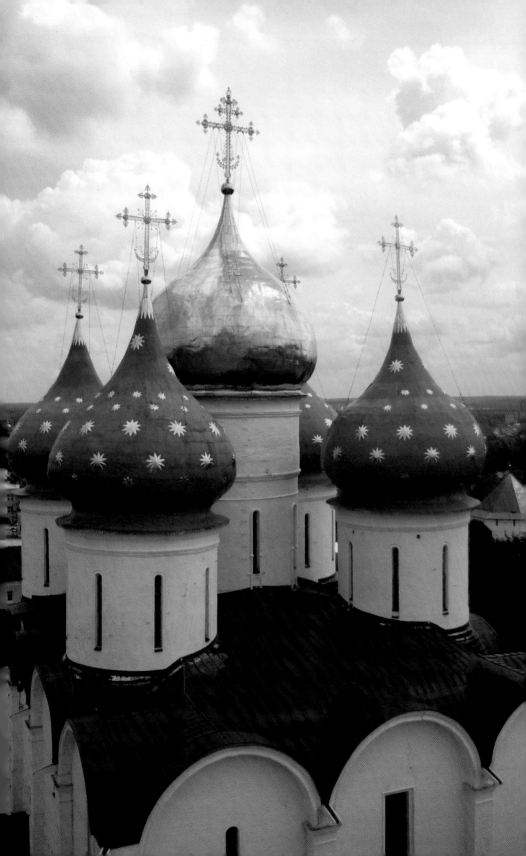

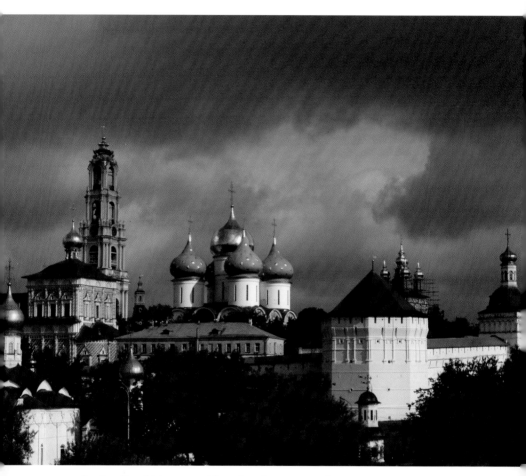
Sergiyev Posad Monastery. (Photo by John A. McGuckin)

translated more often than *The Ladder of Divine Ascent*." Every Lent in every Orthodox monastery it is read aloud as the monks eat their meals. It is also a bestseller among the Orthodox laity throughout the world.

St. John was writing for monks, yet the great popularity of *The Ladder* tells us that men and women living in the world, with families to raise, careers to pursue, and bills to pay, have found in this handbook wisdom that they can borrow to create, as it were, a tiny private monastery of their own where they can be still and commune with God. "Close the door of your cell physically," St. John writes, "the door of your tongue to speech, and the inward door to the evil spirits." Then John offers lay Christians advice on how to grow in holiness in a busy world: "Do whatever good you may," he advises. "Speak evil of no one. Rob no one. Tell no lie. Despise no one. . . . Show compassion to the needy. . . . If you do all this, you will not be far from the kingdom of heaven."

St. John's ladder consists of thirty rungs, or stages in spiritual development (the number thirty corresponding to the age of Jesus when he began his public ministry). Each step up the ladder brings the soul closer to Jesus Christ, who waits at the top, beside a door that leads into heaven. Angels are present along the way to help, but so are demons who try to drag down the climber. The climber's greatest defense against these attacks is constant prayer, repeating the holy name of Jesus, so that he or she is always in the Divine Presence. At one point St. John encourages his readers/climbers, "What higher good is there than to cling to the Lord and persevere in unceasing union with him?"

Beginning the ascent of St. John's ladder is an act of confidence in God. Bishop Kallistos tells us that in the Orthodox Church the first step toward creating a relationship with God is not an examination of conscience and a confession of sins—as is the case in the Catholic Church; rather, the beginner lifts his or her eyes to the glory of God. That is why, the bishop says in *The Orthodox Way*, the Divine Liturgy begins, "Blessed is the kingdom of Father, Son, and Holy Spirit!" A relationship with God begins in hope; there is time for contrition later.

What Is Prayer?

Invariably, when St. John Climacus writes of prayer, he addresses it from a practical perspective. Let your prayers be brief and simple, he says; the prodigal son and the good thief crucified with Jesus offered up one short statement of repentance and they were forgiven. Do not strive for eloquence; searching for the correct term or phrase will just distract you from your purpose. Finally, St. John advises us to be patient: learning to pray without ceasing is comparable to learning how to walk; we will stumble and fall, but if we persist, we will succeed.

For all his pragmatism, there is a point in *The Ladder of Divine Ascent* when St. John appears to have been caught up in a mystical moment as he contemplates the mystery of prayer:

Prayer is the mother and daughter of tears. It is an expiation of sin, a bridge across temptation, a bulwark against affliction. It wipes out conflict, is the work of angels, and is the nourishment of all bodiless beings. Prayer is future gladness, action without end, wellspring of virtues, source of grace, hidden progress, food of the soul, enlightenment of the mind, an axe against despair, hope demonstrated, sorrow done away with.

Encounters with God

Can a human being truly have a direct experience of God—be in some sense in union with God, or perhaps even *see* God? That is a central question of Christian theology, and the various denominations (as well as theologians within those denominations) answer the question in a variety of ways. For Eastern Orthodox ascetics the answer is simple: God can be known and encountered through the Jesus Prayer. Retiring to a silent place, making still all the noise that our ego generates, is essential to preparing for such an experience, but so is cultivating an attitude of being open, of being prepared to listen to the voice of God. When monks or nuns contemplate God through prayer and practice and begin to deeply appreciate the many interventions and compassions of grace offered, their eyes are sometimes filled with tears of joy but also of regret, for in order to live for God alone, they have sacrificed a life with family and friends in the outside world.

Yet even when they have an experience of God, ascetics find it nearly impossible to describe what God is. Such terms as the One, the Supreme Good, the Everlasting Father, and the Creator all fail to convey the essence of God. Like the mystics, we use these terms for God because they suggest his excellence and absolute perfection, but they fall far short just the same. In the end, the one thing we know about God is that he is unknowable. What the mystics experience in the Jesus Prayer is only a glimpse, or perhaps a shadow, of what God truly is.

For thousands of years Jews and Christians have sought God—and found him—in the desert. In the Sinai desert God spoke to Moses from the burning bush, commanding him to lead the Hebrew slaves out of Egypt and into the freedom of the Promised Land. Later, it was on Mount Sinai that God gave Moses the Ten Commandments. In the desert near the Jordan River St. John the Baptist preached repentance and baptism because the Messiah was at hand. And so, following in the footsteps of these prophets and saints, the first Christian hermits and monks traveled deep into the desert in search of God.

The word "desert" comes from the Latin term *desertum,* which means "something left waste"; it is related to the Latin verb *deserere,* "to leave, or forsake." The Greek word for desert is *eremos,* which means "abandonment." From *eremos* we get our English word "hermit."

The desert can be a frightening place: it is vast and devoid of life. Who can exist all alone amid sand and rock, with little or no water, in the inhuman heat of day and the freezing cold of night? Yet both the Bible and the lives of the saints assure us that God drew desperate people to the desert and appeared to them, assuring them that in the wilderness they would be liberated from worldly cares, discover the limitations of human existence, and draw into closer union with

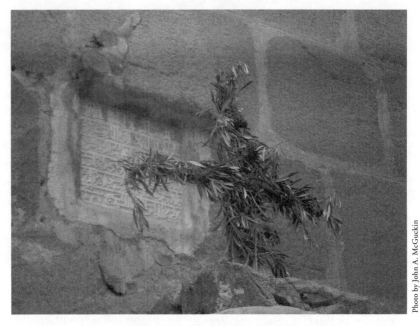

Photo by John A. McGuckin

Cross outside the entrance of St. Catherine's Monastery.

him. Countless holy men and women have borne witness that in the desert, once they had surrendered pride and ego, they did experience extraordinary, indescribable encounters with God.

Of course, not all monasteries and convents are in sandy wastelands. You can find them amid the splendors of the Alps, on bluffs overlooking the Rhine, in the lush meadows of the Ukraine or France or England—or, for that matter, in Iowa, with its beautiful plains and forests. In the case of these monasteries, "desert" has come to mean "remote," or "off the beaten track." Pilgrims and visitors have always made the effort to reach even the most remote monastic houses, and so the monks and nuns have created a kind of desert within their desert—the cloister, the interior of the monastery where (under ordinary circumstances) only the members of the religious community are permitted. Some religious orders, such as the Carthusians, withdraw even from their fellow monks, spending most of their days in solitude in their little houses, working and praying alone with God.

The Carthusians serve as an excellent example for all of us who practice the Jesus Prayer but cannot renounce the world. Find a disused room in your house or a quiet corner of your garden and make it your "desert," where you can go to be alone with God.

In Cairo we met Bishop Youannes, the current general bishop and general secretary to His Holiness Pope Shenouda III, the patriarch of the Coptic Orthodox Church. The bishop addressed this point directly: "Of course, every person in the world needs the calmness of the desert, not only the monks or the nuns . . . because in the crowdedness of the world we don't see ourselves, and we don't see God. But when we [are] in a calmness, especially in the holy places, we begin to look to ourselves, to look to our shortages, to look to our faults, to look to the deepness of our relation with God. To feel God, to hear God."

"The Emperor of Our Peace"

The monks and nuns of previous centuries all agreed that an essential component of beginning a life of prayer was *metanoia,* a Greek term which is usually translated as "change of heart" or "repentance." Father John McGuckin claims that these translations fall short of the mark: *metanoia* is best translated, he says, as "the act of becoming authentic." We become authentic by surrendering our ego to God— admitting our flaws, failings, and sins—and thereby wiping the slate clean, as it were, before beginning a life of prayer and contemplation that will lead us to communion with God.

At Brâncoveanu Monastery in the forests of Transylvania a starets, or spiritual master, spoke to us about the power of prayer. When we pray, Father Teofil said, we "are making a house for him in our heart," and when God enters he brings sublime peace with him. Once united to God, we are never alone, and we need never fear anything again. God becomes our protector, the foundation for our whole life. Suddenly, as he spoke the starets offered a spontaneous prayer of praise: "You are all, God. You are the emperor of our peace and our souls. You are holy and wholly our God. For you are our holiness. For yours is to save and have mercy on us. For you are a God of mercy and of love for humankind."

The starets recalled when he first entered the monastic life and began to recite the Jesus Prayer: "When I started saying, 'Jesus Christ, Son of God,' I . . . actually met the [dirt] of my own soul, and I was frightened," he said. "I couldn't imagine that in my soul one could find so much wickedness, so much bad loathing, which I wouldn't expect to find in my soul. And I wouldn't even make myself conscious that I have it, if I didn't look after my soul through the engagement in prayer. I always tell the people whom I recommend to say this prayer not to get frightened when they discover how much dirt is in their own souls, which should be eliminated, and which does not vanish all of a sudden."

These "terrors of the soul," as the starets described them, can discourage beginners from continuing the practice of the Jesus Prayer. At this crucial moment it is essential for the beginner to press on, to

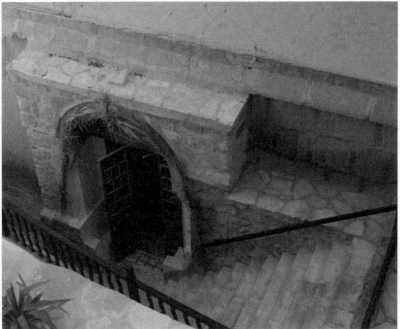

Entrance to the Church of the Transfiguration at St. Catherine's Monastery.

admit one's deepest failings but continue to pray, all the while placing one's trust in the boundless love of Jesus Christ.

The Heart of God

When we were visiting St. Antony's Monastery in Egypt, Father Ruwais pointed out to us that the Arabic word for prayer is *salah,* which means "to make a connection."

"*Salah,* the most expressive word in Arabic, means touching or conducting something or connecting with someone . . . with God," Father Ruwais said. "In English [prayer] means pleading, or asking for something." It is a profound observation that goes to the heart of what we long for in the Jesus Prayer—not to ask something from God, but to make a connection with him.

It was during that visit that Father Lazarus spoke to us at length about his experience of the Jesus Prayer:

"The Jesus Prayer is the heart of God," he said, "and in this you find silence because you have stilled all your passions.

"The Jesus Prayer is, 'Lord Jesus Christ, have mercy on me,' or 'Lord Jesus Christ, Son of God, have mercy on me, a sinner.' That's the short form or the long form—either one, it doesn't matter.

"This prayer starts to diminish—not accelerate—your thoughts. For example, when you pray the Jesus Prayer with concentration, with attention, with love, with humility, with penitence, God graces you with a quiet, peaceful mind.

" 'Lord.' You have to acknowledge that you are saying something when you are saying Lord.

" 'Jesus.' There is no other name by which you can be saved. He is the Savior.

" 'Christ.' He's the Anointed One. God anointed him; God made him the One to save us.

" 'Lord Jesus Christ.' You already have a whole theology in only three words.

"So if you are breathing, 'Lord Jesus Christ,' you take in, you breathe in with your breath the name of the Lord; you hold it and

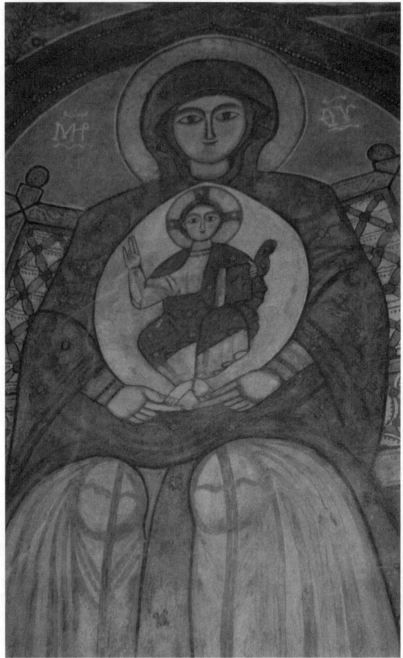

A thirteenth-century icon of the Holy Virgin Mary and Christ painted
on the wall of the St. Antony Church, St. Antony's Monastery.

take God into yourself. When you confess your sins, when you confess as Peter confessed, 'You are the Lord,' then you confess your sins, 'have mercy on me'; you breathe them out.

"This is a marriage of body and soul. This is a purification of your body by your prayer. It is already an accelerated way of silence because you arrive at a point where your mind is still because it's surrendered to Jesus."

Transforming Solitude into Communion

The quest for fulfillment and inner peace is old and ongoing. I found this desire to be fundamental to the life of the monks and nuns in all the monastic communities we visited. It came as a bit of a surprise to discover that they believed that such peace was not limited to monastics, but could also be attained (to some degree at least) in the outside world. In fact, a recurring theme of the conversations I had with many monks and nuns was their contention that the Jesus Prayer has the power to purge what is superficial and connect people with God. The Jesus Prayer, they told me, can cure the ills of urban and suburban modernity, reuniting people, freeing them from self-inflicted isolation, from overconsumption, and reveal to them a vision of life that is more than the accumulation of ever more expensive stuff. The practice of the Jesus Prayer, of contemplation in silence—whether in the stillness of nature or in a sacred place, at home or at work—has the power to revive and repair the inner self, helping to restore a person to creative expression and profound peace, and opening up the mind and heart, perhaps for the first time, to what it means to be fully alive. This is what I observed and experienced at these ancient and still very much alive holy sites.

As noted earlier, this point was made by Bishop Daniel Ciobotea, who at the time was metropolitan of Moldavia and Bukovina and is now patriarch of the Romanian Orthodox Church. "Today some great cities, big cities—*megalopolises*—are similar to the desert," he said, "not because there are not many people in them, but certain similarity is given by the feeling of solitude. Although there are crowds of

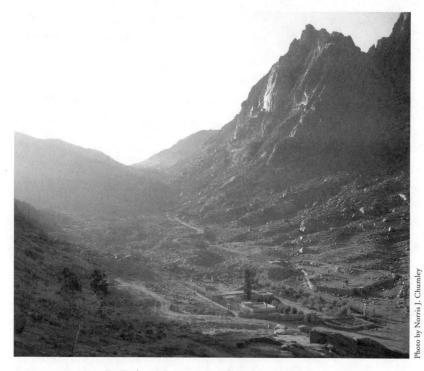

Photo by Norris J. Chumley

St. Catherine's Monastery from Mount Horeb,
with the sun rising behind Mount Sinai.

people, many persons are feeling like [they are] in the desert because there is not enough communion, not enough communication, and I think the [Jesus] Prayer is to transform the solitude into communion, and first of all communion with God, fellowship with God."

This is an insightful reimagining of the concept of the desert. What the bishop was saying is that many of us are already living in desert-like isolation even though we live in big cities or towns with many people. Our apartments, our houses have become our cells into which we retreat, living enclosed lives entirely cut off from our neighbors, who themselves are living exactly the same way. Why not, then, transform our isolation into contemplation and prayer and make a connection with God? Why not join in fellowship with others who are seeking spiritual revelation and transformation, seeking reconciliation and redemption through Christ? That's how the first monastic communities were founded. The cities may become the new desert, and the gathering of practitioners of the Jesus Prayer the new monks and nuns.

When I asked the bishop what we could do to experience God in the context of our day-to-day lives as ordinary, secular people, he said, "What is important is to be united with God. . . . The important attitude is to remind us that we are in the presence of God. And to start to speak with him silently, not just by words. And this communion of our mind with God, it's the beginning of a good prayer, although we are in the cities, or we are working in the office. And it's a question of desire to meet God and to let God share in our life. And in this sense we can conclude then to say that prayer is not only *our* activity; it is the activity also of God in us."

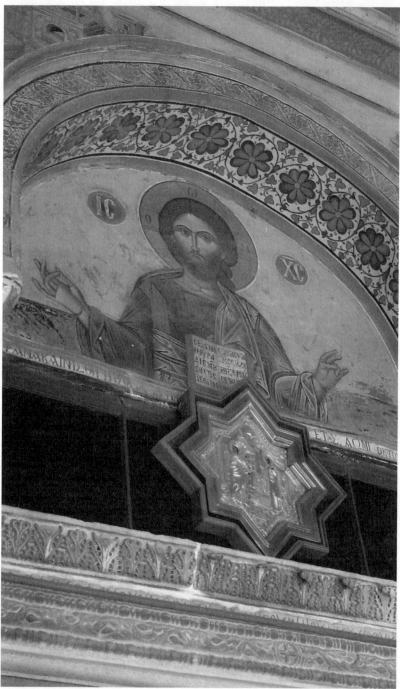

4

The Jesus Prayer on the Holy Mountain

The Monasteries of Mount Athos

T HERE WE WERE, FACE TO FACE. All my best-intentioned plans, not to mention my nervousness and insecurities, dissolved as I kissed the hand of the black-robed, long-bearded man. Abbot Ephraim, the archimandrite (or head) of Vatopedi, the second-largest monastery on Mount Athos, also called the Holy Mountain, smiled a welcoming grin. His eyes were warm and kind as, in truncated English, he said, "So you are one who makes this film about us?"

"Yes," I replied. "Your blessing, please, Father. We've come from America. I love God, and I want to help other people find God with this film and book we are making on the heart of the monastic life."

Father John had trained me in all the proper signs and terms of respect: kissing the hand, using proper titles, mentioning that I am a follower of Christ and "a student of matters of the soul." The abbot

---

Opposite: An exterior icon of Christ, over the main door to the *katholikon* at Vatopedi Monastery on Mount Athos.

chuckled after I made my introduction, looking at his three assistants, who chuckled with him. Despite that suggestion of good humor, in the silence that followed I felt nervous again. Being a producer from way back, I didn't allow my nerves to get the best of me, however—at least not yet. I knew I was asking a lot of the monks. Filming of any kind is prohibited on Mount Athos, and visitors can't even bring in still cameras. Photographing monks is forbidden; even photographing the monasteries they live in is forbidden.

There are rules upon rules on Mount Athos, dating back a thousand years. No women allowed on the peninsula from which the Holy Mountain arises; no non-Orthodox permitted in the monastery churches; no non-Orthodox allowed to receive the Eucharist; no non-Orthodox invited to dine with the monks.

In spite of these restrictions, the visitors—pilgrims, officially—keep coming, so the monks on Athos have taken steps to limit the ever-increasing throngs of intruders, people like us. The regulations in force at Vatopedi at the time of my stay limited non-Orthodox

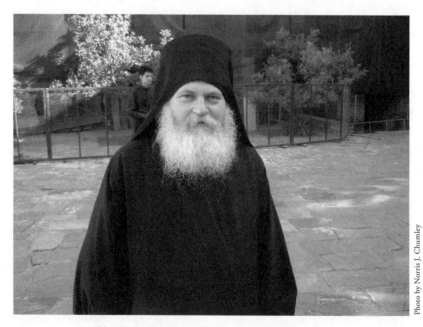

Photo by Norris J. Chumley

Abbot Ephraim, Vatopedi Monastery, Mount Athos.

visitors to four per day, and Orthodox visitors to a hundred per day. Such measures may strike some as stingy, but from the monks' point of view these strictures are absolutely necessary in order to preserve their traditions and, most importantly, their life of prayer in an atmosphere of solitude and silence. It occurred to me that day that the last thing the monks might want would be a film producer whose documentary would cast a spotlight on their Holy Mountain and attract even larger crowds of pilgrims.

Before Abbot Ephraim changed his mind and showed me the door, I put on my producer hat and, speaking perhaps a little too quickly, explained how I'd received special permission in advance from the country's two patriarchs to bring an assistant, a camera, and recording equipment to Mount Athos. As I opened my bag to show my equipment to him, Abbot Ephraim shook his head and backed away from me, as if I were about to draw out something unholy, or at least unwholesome. The abbot's assistants were all aflutter, shaking their heads as well. I reached into the bag for my letter from one of the patriarchs, but thought better of it and left it where it lay.

With a slight gesture of his hand Abbot Ephraim motioned for everyone to calm down, and the tension broke. Once again he looked into my eyes, then patted me on my chest, over my heart. I could feel a powerful energy coursing from my head to my toes. He smiled again and said, "Fine. You are sincere." It felt as if he'd psychically read my soul, examined my intentions, and I had passed. Then the abbot asked, "This first time to the Holy Mountain?"

"Yes," I said, "but I have been here in my dreams and prayers many times." The monks all smiled, and I could feel that they loved hearing this. The main assistant, an old monk, addressed me: "Father says you may take pictures anywhere, and make sound recordings."

"In the church?" I asked. I could scarcely believe my luck. "Anywhere? Everywhere? And the monks?"

The abbot nodded affirmatively while the older assistant added, "The Holy Council forbids *filming;* we can't change that." This sentiment was echoed by Abbot Ephraim's nods. "You may make lots of beautiful pictures and sounds, though, with our blessings."

They would have let me shoot video, I thought, if the mountain community hadn't forbidden it. I was happy just to be allowed to stay, and to make unlimited stills and sound recordings, and I was delighted that I'd won the abbot's confidence so quickly. Give me a centimeter and I'll ask for a kilometer, though, so I decided to request a little more: "May I please have an interview with Father?"

Abbot Ephraim himself said, "Yes. We will work on that." Then the elderly assistant took me by the hand and escorted me out of the monastery's offices.

"Thank you. Thank you. God bless you, Father," I said as he led us out. I looked at my assistant, Todd Lester, who looked as amazed as I was. We were *in*. We were inside the inside, at the very heart of monastic practice—inside the great, mystical Mount Athos.

Squabbling Monks and Hermits

Mount Athos rises from a rugged, heavily forested peninsula in north-eastern Greece that measures 37 miles long and 7.5 miles wide and covers an area of about 217 square miles. The mountain itself soars to a height of 6,670 feet. Scattered across the peninsula, hidden away in the forests, are twenty monasteries and about as many sketes, or small communities of hermits (that is, hermitages).

There have been monks on Mount Athos since the fifth century, but the story of the Holy Mountain as we see it today begins in the mid-tenth century with the friendship of the monk St. Athanasios and the Byzantine emperor Nicephorus Phocas. In 963, supplied with funds from the emperor, Athanasios began building the first of Athos's major monasteries, the Great Lavra. Among his other gifts to the Great Lavra, Nicephorus donated a large Bible, its cover studded with jewels, and a golden reliquary containing a portion of the true Cross of Jesus; both of these treasures are still in the possession of the monks of the Great Lavra. Many of the hermits who lived on the mountain rejected the idea of leaving their dank caves and tiny huts to move into the monastery, and so to this day the monks of Mount

Athos have their choice of living in community within a monastery or living in solitude in the forest.

The harmony that exists today between the monks and the hermits took years to achieve. The unseemly squabbling over which was the holier way of life raged on Mount Athos for a decade, outliving even the Great Lavra's patron, Nicephorus (who, by the way, at the end of his life abdicated and spent his final years as a monk at the monastery). In 972 the new emperor, John Tzimiskes, sent Abbot Euthymios of the Studion Monastery in Constantinople to Athos to serve as mediator. The outcome of Euthymios's arbitration was a 972 charter known as the Tragos (from the Greek word for "goat," because the parchment was made from a goat's skin). The Tragos, among other things, guaranteed the independence of the hermits from the authority of the monks and established an assembly comprising monks and hermits to govern the peninsula. Both Emperor John Tzimiskes and Athanasios signed the charter, which is preserved in the archives of the town of Karyes, the administrative center of the Holy Mountain. In later centuries Mount Athos was recognized in the Byzantine Empire as an independent monastic republic. Today Mount Athos is a self-governing part of Greece.

The Garden of the Virgin Mary

An old and venerable tradition claims that after Jesus Christ ascended into heaven, the Virgin Mary and St. John the Apostle sailed to Cyprus to visit Lazarus, the man Christ had raised from the dead, who was now bishop of the island. A storm at sea forced Our Lady and the Beloved Disciple to shelter in a bay at the foot of Mount Athos, near the spot where the Monastery of Iviron stands today. Delighted by the beauty of the mountain, Mary asked her Son to give it to her, and Jesus acquiesced. "Let this place be your lot," he may have said, "your garden and your paradise, as well as a salvation, a haven for those who seek salvation." Ever since, Mount Athos has been known as the Garden of the Virgin Mary.

There is a holy icon of Mary at Iviron, which is highly venerated and a living reminder that Athos and everyone who lives there belongs, in a unique way, to the Mother of Christ. After I had seen the icon, a novice monk of Iviron confided to me that he thought the legend wasn't true: he doubted that the Virgin herself had ever set foot on Mount Athos. He was glad, though, that women weren't allowed on Athos because, he confessed to me, back in the world he'd had "girlfriend problems" and was happy to be away from them.

Traditionally monks from across the Orthodox nations of Europe—Greece, Russia, Serbia, Bulgaria, Georgia, Romania—were drawn to Athos. Today, Orthodox men come from as far away as Africa, the United States, and Peru to discern their vocation in the monasteries. These new monks have revived monastic life on the Holy Mountain. In the 1960s it seemed that Athos was dying. There were about 1,100 monks in residence, and their median age was roughly fifty-five. Today there are approximately 2,200 monks on Mount Athos, and most of the novices are in their twenties or thirties.

The new monks are men of the twentieth and twenty-first centuries. Many of them have university degrees, and all have modern skills that are being put to good use. For the first time in history, the manuscripts, icons, liturgical vestments, and sacred vessels of the Mount Athos monasteries are being catalogued. One outcome of that project was a blockbuster museum exhibition, "The Treasures of Mount Athos," which went on display at the Museum of Byzantine Culture in Thessaloniki in 1997. It was the first time these extraordinary works of art had ever been seen outside the Holy Mountain.

In virtually every other respect, however, the new monks follow a way of life that has barely changed in a thousand years. The Byzantine day begins with vespers (*esperinos*), which lasts from the late afternoon until sunset. This is followed by a light meal for supper, then the service of compline (*apodeipnon*), and finally a little time for relaxation before the monks retire to their cells. After several hours of sleep, the monks are up at three in the morning and start their day with the morning office (*orthros*), a church service that anticipates sunrise. Morning prayer concludes with the highest moment of the day, the Divine Liturgy, and communion with God in the form of Holy Communion—the partaking of consecrated bread and wine, which is the Body and Blood of Christ. Following the Divine Liturgy the main meal is served to the priests, monks, and pilgrims. From one until three in the afternoon the monks perform some kind of labor before returning to the church for vespers, which begins the cycle once again.

"Appeal to the Lord Quietly"

Mount Athos has been a cradle of saints, but in terms of the Jesus Prayer certainly one of the most influential has been St. Gregory of Sinai. He was born about the year 1265 on the Aegean coast in what is now Turkey. As a boy, Gregory, his entire family, and almost all of their fellow villagers were taken captive by Turkish pirates and held for ransom. Once they had all been delivered from that danger, Gregory, although probably barely in his teens, chose not to return home but traveled instead to Cyprus to begin his formation as a monk. After his novitiate on Cyprus he went to Mount Sinai, to the Monastery of St. Catherine, where he made his solemn profession of monastic vows. A few years later Gregory was on the move again, this time to Crete, where he placed himself under the guidance of a monk named Arsenios, a man steeped in the art of contemplative prayer. It was Arsenios who taught Gregory how to make the Jesus Prayer an active, ongoing interior conversation with God.

From Crete Gregory, now about thirty-five years old, went to Mount Athos, where he settled in a skete called Magoula near the Philotheou Monastery. Some ruins of Magoula still stand. It is said that Gregory found on Athos only three monks who practiced contemplative prayer, and so he set about renewing the spiritual life on the Holy Mountain by restoring the ancient practice—specifically, through the Jesus Prayer. He promised the monks that if they said the Jesus Prayer silently without ceasing, they would experience in a dynamic way "the energy of the Holy Spirit, which we have already mystically received in baptism."

In his work *Instructions to the Hesychasts,* also known as *On Stillness and Prayer,* Gregory advises anyone who sets out to say the Jesus Prayer aloud to "appeal to the Lord quietly and without agitation, so that the voice does not disturb the attention of the mind and does not thus break off the prayer, until the mind is accustomed to this . . . and, receiving force from the Spirit, firmly prays within on its own. Then there will be no need to say the prayer with the lips."

Of course, Gregory was conscious of the unbidden distractions that enter the mind even during the most intense moments of concentration. In his *Instructions to the Hesychasts,* he says "When you notice thoughts arising and accosting you," he said, "do not look at them, even if they are not bad; but keeping the mind firmly in the heart, call to Lord Jesus and you will soon sweep away the thoughts and drive out their instigators—the demons."

Ever a restless soul, Gregory did not stay on Mount Athos, but spent the last years of his life in the Strandzha Mountains in Bulgaria. He died there in 1346.

During my visit to Mount Athos, Abbot Ephraim spoke to me about his own mentor and spiritual father, Elder Joseph (1898–1959), who had learned to detach himself from worldly things so completely that his entire life was dedicated to communion with God. As he achieved complete inner stillness, the recitation of the Jesus Prayer became constant and automatic, which is the goal of every monk and nun.

Twenty Permission Requests

Getting onto the Holy Mountain is not for the faint-hearted, and it is certainly not for a mere tourist. Potential guests must be seriously determined. The monks require every visitor, whether Orthodox or not, to have a visitation permit known as a *diamoneterion,* which is valid for only four calendar days. Getting a permit sounds easy, but the *diamoneterion* is one of the most bureaucracy-laden documents I've ever attempted to acquire.

I began by writing and faxing and calling and meeting with every influential Greek Orthodox priest and church authority I could find in America, and I corresponded with many in Greece as well. I tried going through arts councils, government offices, friends who knew influential people (who themselves knew even more influential people). Repeatedly I called and emailed Bob Allison, the head of the Friends of Mount Athos organization in the United States. Finally, Father Robert Stephanopoulos, head of communications for the Greek Orthodox Church in the United States, and his wife, Nikki (parents of the newscaster and political commentator George Stephanopoulos), tried to expedite the matter for me by asking a blessing on my film project from His Eminence Archbishop Demetrios, the primate of the Greek Orthodox Church in America. His Eminence did indeed bless us and the movie, and he then did me the tremendous favor of requesting an additional blessing from His All Holiness Ecumenical Patriarch Bartholomew of Constantinople (Istanbul).

Two months later, unexpectedly in the morning's mail, came a hand-inscribed letter from His All Holiness, written in the archaic formal Greek used by the Greek Orthodox Church. I was thrilled, but of course I couldn't read it. Father John promptly supplied a translation, which informed us that we had the blessing of the patriarch, which was in essence a guarantee that we would receive a *diamoneterion* for Mount Athos. In the midst of our excitement Father John warned me that the Athonite monks are unswervingly Orthodox, committed to preserving their ancient faith and traditions no matter what. I didn't completely understand all that Father John's warning entailed, as I would soon discover.

I faxed the patriarch's letter to the Pilgrim Bureau in both Thessaloniki and Ouranoupolis, the closest mainland town to the Athos Peninsula, requesting a *diamoneterion*. No answer. Undaunted, I telephoned. The monks speak very few words of English, and my Greek is limited to "love God" = *agape Theo*, "visit" = *episcopse*, and "film" = *photographo*. None of these words did any good.

After five fruitless international calls, at last the phone at the Holy Mountain's administrative center in Karyes was handed to a monk named Alix, who was fluent in English. I made my request again, this time with more hope of success. He instructed me to write and fax another letter. I did so promptly, and three weeks later a letter of permission to enter the Holy Mountain arrived by fax. Unfortunately, it emphatically and explicitly denied permission to film.

Reluctantly, I began making phone calls to Mount Athos again. About ten calls later I got Alix on the phone. He gave me verbal permission to bring a camera and directed me to mention his name when I arrived, but he cautioned that I still had obstacles to overcome. Every monastery on Athos is an independent entity, he warned; if the abbot of Monastery A gave me permission to take photos of his monastery, the abbot of Monastery B would be under no obligation to follow suit. With twenty monasteries on the Holy Mountain, I would be obliged to file twenty permission requests!

And there was another matter: overnight accommodations. Pilgrims and visitors who intend to stay on Mount Athos overnight must make advance reservations. "This will be almost impossible during the summer, when many pilgrims come," Alix said. "You should have done this a year ago."

The trip was only three weeks away. With nonrefundable plane tickets in hand, I wasn't about to give up. I obtained the fax and phone numbers for the twenty monasteries and began my double campaign to obtain permission to photograph and to reserve a room in a monastery guesthouse for me and my assistant.

The monks open their offices for only a couple of hours a day, between prayers and church services, and they only occasionally answer phones and faxes, preferring to preserve their isolation from the world as much as possible. Of course, no one I reached at any of the various monasteries spoke English, and my Greek was so terrible that the person on the other end would hang up on me impatiently. Finally, persistence got me someone who did speak a little English—a monk at Vatopedi. He gave us a room, but for only two nights. So what about the other two nights? We'd figure that out later.

The Journey to Mount Athos

In our tiny rental car, we dashed from Athens to Ouranoupolis to get the one daily boat for Mount Athos, which leaves precisely at 9:30 A.M. Ouranoupolis, which means "City of the Heavens," is a beautiful little beach town. Initially it struck me as odd that the overwhelming majority of sunbathers I saw lounging on the beach were women. Then I realized—these were the mothers, wives, and daughters of the pilgrims; they would wait here while the menfolk of their families spent several days in prayer and contemplation on the Holy Mountain.

We joined the men waiting in line to buy tickets for the boat to Daphni, Mount Athos's main port. Surprisingly, the security guard

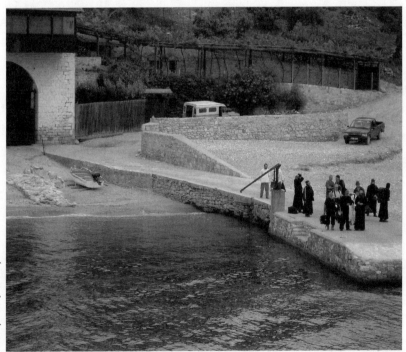

One of the points of arrival to the Holy Mountain, Mount Athos,
where the monks await the daily ferry to the mainland.

who was checking bags let us right on the ferry with three bags full of cameras and high-tech audio gear—no questions asked.

The boat was jam-packed with brusque men, mostly Greek laymen, and about a dozen monks carrying loaves of bread and plastic bags of odds and ends from the outer world. We, with our American clothes and hats, were obviously the foreigners. No one spoke to us or even acknowledged that we were there. As the boat eased away from its anchorage I watched the monks throw crusts of bread off the starboard side to seagulls.

About two hours into the trip, with only sea in view, we spotted a completely green, mountainous wilderness. This must be Mount Athos, I thought. It looked primal and very isolated, with wind-shaped trees and forbidding rock cliffs. Suddenly a man next to us belted out, "That's Prodromos, the Romanian monastery. See the pier? That's where I'm going." Then, pointing to another cluster of buildings, he said, "There's the Russian monastery, St. Panteleimon." We struck up a conversation with him about the different monasteries

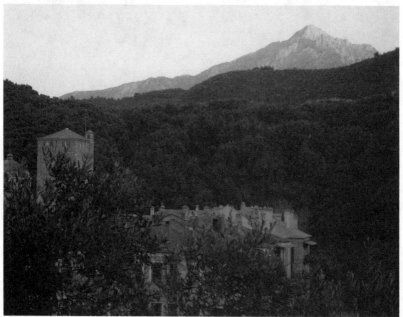

Mount Athos, the Holy Mountain.

Photo by Norris J. Chumley

and the history of the Holy Mountain. He'd been there many times, he said, but not to Vatopedi, where we were headed.

At the tiny pier at Daphni we stood aside politely as the pilgrims stampeded down the dock to get a seat on a bus. We were so polite we almost didn't make it onto what was the only shuttle from Daphni to the main town of Karyes. As it was, we were obliged to stand for the whole bumpy forty-five-minute ride. This was followed by standing for another hour in at least hundred-degree heat on Karyes's Holy Ghost Street, waiting for a minivan that would take us to Vatopedi.

After a wild ride to the monastery, with the van careening up dirt roads and along excruciatingly narrow mountain paths, we arrived at the gate to Vatopedi.

"No. Ris. Ch- Ch- Chumumley," the gatekeeper called out. "Who is he?"

I gulped, said "Here," and raised my hand.

"Oh . . . oh . . . yes, reservation for two in your name." He raised the barrier outside the gate and we were in. Thank God again.

Living in Byzantine Time

Vatopedi, part monastery, part stronghold, has the look of a medieval fortress and sits high on a hill overlooking the Aegean Sea, surrounded by a magnificent ten-story brick wall. As we passed through the entryway, through the thick monastery wall, I glanced up and saw stunning murals of Jesus and Mary painted on the ceiling. Men driving oxcarts piled high with hand-chiseled building stones rolled along the narrow cobblestone roadway past the front gate. Monks trooped by in black cassocks. No one stopped to greet us. The gatekeeper, Father Paul, peeked out a window, checked our papers for a long while, then, emerging from his post, welcomed us to Vatopedi.

We were shown to our *archontariki,* or guesthouse (one of several), led up a set of rickety stairs and into a long hallway where stood a long, bare table. After a few minutes, a priest about my age with two young boys came in and sat down, followed by the *archontaris,* the guesthouse master. They served us Greek coffee in delicate porcelain

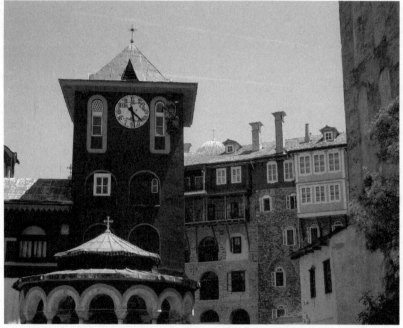

A side view from the courtyard of Vatopedi Monastery on Mount Athos. This shows the clock tower and part of the main church, over ten centuries old.

cups, small glasses of what I took to be water, and white-powdered candies. I took a drink of the water and nearly choked. It was raki, a sharp alcoholic drink that tastes of fennel and turpentine. Nonetheless, after the shock of the first sip, I found it curiously delicious.

The *archontaris* explained the monastery's regulations for pilgrims. We were to attend all church services beginning that day at five, and then tomorrow at three . . . in the morning. Todd and I looked at each other, trying to conceal our dismay over getting up so early. Earlier Todd had said he'd join me around eight or nine, which had sounded good to me!

That's when I noticed the large picture of the Theotokos, the Holy Mother of God, hanging on a wall between two clocks, each showing different times. "Why two?" I asked, and pointed.

One of the monks replied, "Byzantine time. Forget about it; it's impossible for you to follow."

Vatopedi is extremely photogenic, despite the fact that at the time of our visit a quarter of the complex was shrouded under scaffolding, in the midst of an ambitious renovation project funded in large part by England's Prince Charles. Almost from the moment we arrived, Todd and I began taking what would ultimately tally up to 500 photographs: the Vatopedi monks, the church, the dozens of chapels, the monks' cells, the guesthouses, the stone walks, the suspended walkways, the plazas paved with ancient slates, the kitchen, the workshops—in other words, an entire town contained within the walls of a tenth-century monastery. We also photographed the surrounding fields of meticulously tended vegetables, the groves of fruit and olive trees, the vineyards, and the monks' fishing boats. Vatopedi is a completely self-sustaining community: the monks catch all the fish, grow all the vegetables, and make all the feta cheese and bread they eat.

As for the monastery's location, we found ourselves set down between a beautiful stretch of beach and an untouched mountain

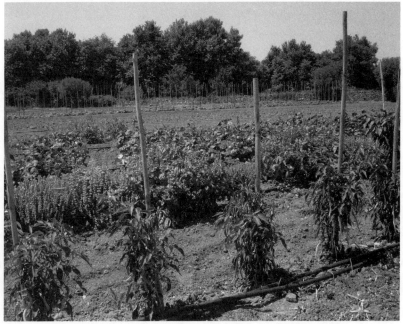

Photo by Norris J. Chumley

Monks' vegetable garden, Vatopedi Monastery, Mount Athos.

wilderness. Nothing else—no hamlets or towns, not a thing man-made—is nearby. And all of Athos is like this: dense forests, huge rocks, mountain paths, and dirt lanes, a place as undisturbed and undeveloped as I've ever seen. The monks have done nothing that might alter the sacred, timeless character of this place.

. . .

One of the traditions that took root on Mount Athos was introduced by St. Gregory Palamas (1296–1359), a monk of Vatopedi who developed a method of reciting the Jesus Prayer that is linked to breathing. Father Ruwais first taught us this at St. Antony's Monastery in Egypt. As the monk inhales, he prays, "Lord Jesus Christ, Son of God," then pauses a moment, holding his breath, before exhaling and praying, "have mercy on me, a sinner." St. Palamas explains, "In this way, [the monk] will also be able to control the mind together with the breath." It is a form of prayer that requires the focus of mind and heart, intellect and body.

St. Palamas's method is known as *hesychasm,* or the practice of stillness. As we saw earlier, this is a type of contemplation in which one focuses body and mind on one goal—unceasing prayer. By entering a monastery or convent, a monk or nun physically withdraws from the noise of the secular world. Through *hesychasm,* he or she then withdraws deeply into him/herself to maintain a constant conversation with God. The inspiration for this private form of prayer is drawn from the Sermon on the Mount as recorded in St. Matthew's Gospel: "But when you pray," Jesus says, "go into your room and shut the door and pray to your Father who is in secret; and your Father who sees in secret will reward you" (Matt. 6:6). The "room" mentioned by Christ is the interior, the soul, the *nous*—that place where the monk or nun becomes aware of the presence of God. It is the constant recitation of the Jesus Prayer that is the monastic's spiritual passport to that secret and sacred place.

Abbot Ephraim spoke of this during our conversation. "For all Christians, especially the monks," he said, "silence is important. But

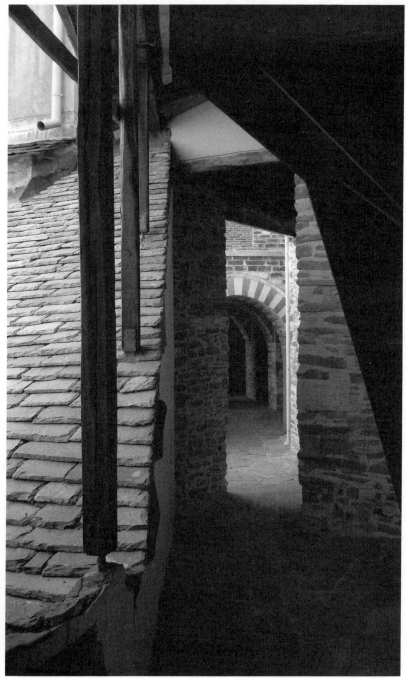

Photo by Norris J. Chumley

Monks' walkway, Vatopedi Monastery, Mount Athos.

this does not mean only, 'Don't speak.' Mainly, silence, from the theological point of view, is the concentration of all the inner powers, in the mind, in the heart, and the inner union of our *nous*. This is the main point of the teaching of St. Gregory Palamas. This can be achieved through the Jesus Prayer."

For St. Palamas *hesychasm* is not one type of prayer among many, but "the whole purpose of Christian life." He believed that the point or goal of Christianity is to purify the heart and enter so deeply into the contemplation of God that God will graciously grant a glimpse of his glory. St. Palamas likened such an experience to the Transfiguration, when Christ took his three favorite apostles, Sts. Peter, James, and John, to the summit of Mount Tabor and there let them see him in his divine splendor. According to St. Palamas, the continual practice of reciting the Jesus Prayer may culminate in the type of vision the three apostles experienced on that mountain.

I don't know how many of the monks on Mount Athos have been granted such a special grace, but I believe that it represents what all of them desire and strive for.

The Communion of Saints

The sound of a *talanton* called us to church. A long board struck by a mallet, the *talanton* is the means by which the monks summon people to prayer and the Divine Liturgy. In ancient times the monks rang a *simantron,* a metal bell, but wave after wave of invasions and conquests had taught the monks to be cautious about attracting attention to themselves. This sense of caution was also the reason for the impenetrable walls of the monastery. Originally built around 972, Vatopedi has withstood multiple attacks from the Turks, pirates, and even Crusaders from western Europe. I wasn't the first to work hard to gain entrance.

It was indeed a harsh awakening to hear the pounding of the *talanton* right outside our door at two-thirty in the morning, but I was determined to go to the morning office in the church. Todd, though, rolled over and went back to sleep. Dragging myself out of bed, I pulled on my clothes, left the guesthouse, and followed cobble-stone walkways to Vatopedi's thousand-year-old *katholikon,* or primary church. I knew it was the custom for non-Orthodox to remain in the narthex, the outer vestibule of the church, but one of the abbot's assistants waved me in, then sat me in the front row, where I had an excellent view of the monks in their choir stalls.

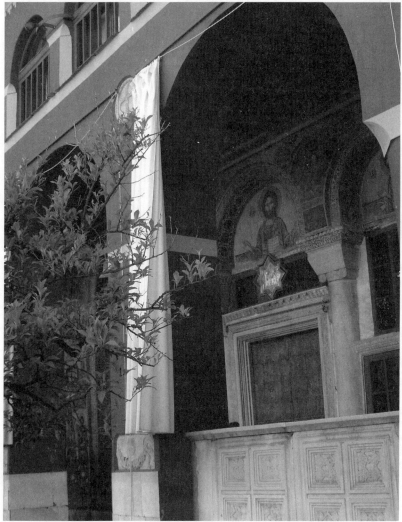

Photo by Norris J. Chumley

Entrance to the *katholikon,* Vatopedi Monastery, Mount Athos.

The darkness of the *katholikon* was broken only where a few candles in brass chandeliers suspended from the ceiling gleamed before some of the icons. Mingled with sounds in the church, from a distant chapel I could hear the voice of a priest as he sang in minor tone a prayer in liturgical Greek; the language was incomprehensible to me, yet it was a transcendent moment.

Millions upon millions of prayers have been offered up in this church for a thousand years. This is a place where a visitor could feel the infinite mystery of Christ's teachings and gifts. As one stands in the dark church witnessing the monks' total love of and devotion to God, the Virgin, the martyrs, the apostles, and all the saints, the Christian doctrine of the "communion of saints" becomes alive.

Following an ancient liturgy that I could barely follow, the monks circled the nave over and over, bowing low to kiss the icons on the iconostasis separating the sanctuary with its altar from the main body of the church. Large icons of Jesus Christ and the Theotokos, Mary the Mother of God, flanked the golden central door, which symbolizes the threshold between heaven and earth. The musky aroma of incense permeated the vast chamber. Glancing up, I took in the domed ceiling, lit by a crown of candles that barely revealed an image of Christ looking down upon us as if from heaven itself.

Then the monks gathered around an ornately carved wooden stand and began to intone various psalms. Their voices were the most beautifully trained I'd ever heard. Like angels they were, singing the praises of God all day and all night.

The music of the chant was familiar to me; I had been to Orthodox services before. I could pick out the word *sophia,* which means "wisdom," and always heralds a reading from the scriptures. *Kyrie eleison,* or "Lord, have mercy," was another phrase I knew. What struck me most, however, was the rhythms of the chant, the cadences of the ancient language, to which inexplicably my intuition and soul became more and more attuned. By putting aside the logical, cerebral understanding of words and language, I had entered into the mystery of the liturgy.

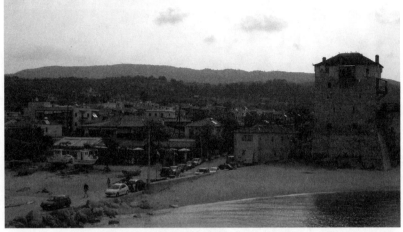

Photo by Norris J. Chumley

The daily ferry sets out from Ouranoupolis (Greek for "City of Heaven")
on the way to the Holy Mountain, Mount Athos.

Then, in my totally relaxed, transcendent moment of spiritual ecstasy—whack! A monk slapped me on the shoulder. I'd fallen peace-
fully asleep, and it was this monk's task to wake anyone who dozed
off during this early-morning service. I'm embarrassed to admit that
the monk had to come back to slap me awake many times. When the
sunrise came, and glowing rays of light streamed through the ancient
stained-glass windows, it was much easier to stay awake. By that time
the monks and I had been in church for four hours.

Another hour went by and the Divine Liturgy was celebrated, cul-
minating with the distribution of the consecrated bread and wine in
Holy Communion. The priests inside the sanctuary received first,
then the other chanting monks, and after them a handful of Orthodox pilgrims who were in the church with me. In the meantime, Todd
had crept in and sat down beside me. As non-Orthodox we could
not receive Communion, and we wondered if it was obvious to the
monks and the congregation that we were not. But given the graces I
had experienced in the church that night, and the permission to take
pictures throughout Vatopedi, that was in a sense enough of a holy
feast for us.

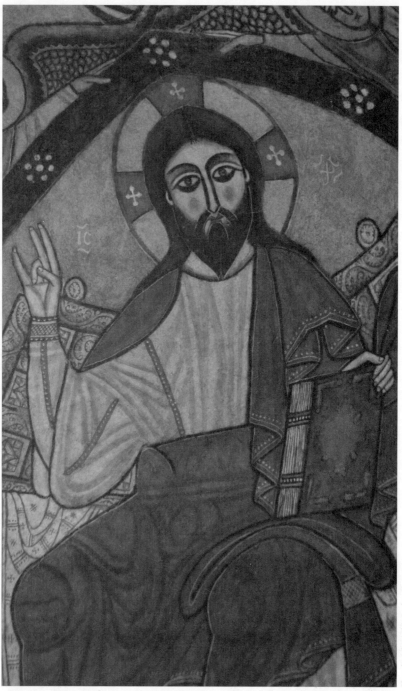

5

The History of the
Jesus Prayer

W HEN JESUS CHRIST came to earth more than 2,000 years
ago, the people of Israel had already developed a profound
reverence for the holy name of God. This name, which God had revealed to Moses, the Jews had come to regard as ineffable, so sacred
that it could not be pronounced even in prayer. In its place, the Jews
adopted the title *Adonai,* "the Lord"; but in time even that seemed too
bold, and so it became customary to refer in Hebrew to God as *Ha
Shem,* which means "the Name." In Jesus's day, the true name of God
was spoken aloud only once a year, on Yom Kippur, the Day of Atone-
ment, when the high priest entered the Holy of Holies in the Temple
of Jerusalem and there, all alone, pronounced the sacred name.

No such prohibitions were ever attached to the name of Jesus.
How could they be? His name had been pronounced by probably
thousands when he was present on earth. Furthermore, in its Hebrew
form, Yeshua (Joshua in English), it was a common name. Even if

---

Opposite: An icon of Christ "Pantocrator" ("Ruler of All") on the ceiling of a tiny
chapel altar in St. Antony Church at St. Antony's Monastery in Egypt. Painted in
the thirteenth century, it has been recently restored.

the first Christians wanted to bar anyone from speaking the name of Jesus, how could they enforce it?

Nonetheless, *reverence* for the name of Jesus dates back to the age of the apostles. In the Gospel of St. John Jesus himself encourages his disciples to draw upon the power of his name: "If you ask anything of the Father, he will give it to you in my name" (John 16:23). Not long afterward St. Paul would write in his letter to the Philippians, "At the name of Jesus every knee should bow, in heaven and on earth and under the earth" (Phil. 2:10).

About the year 150 a Christian mystic known as Hermas wrote down a series of visions he had received; this book is known as *The Shepherd*. During one of these visions an angel assured Hermas, "No one shall enter into the kingdom of God, except he receive the name of His Son." Later the angel tells Hermas, "The name of the Son of God is great and incomprehensible, and sustaineth the whole world."

Here we see that by the second century Christians were developing a theology of the power of the name of Jesus. If, as some believe, the

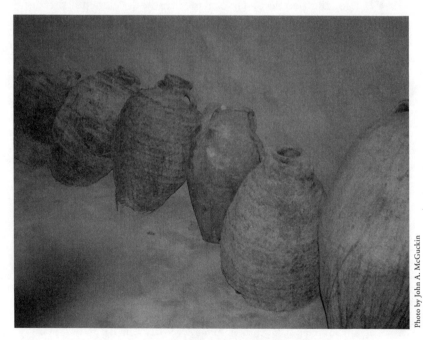

Jugs for water and oil, St. Antony's Monastery.

Photo by John A. McGuckin

Jesus Prayer dates back to the time of Christ, then these lines from *The Shepherd* are expressing an existing religious devotion. But if the Jesus Prayer is of a later date, then we have found one of its earliest forerunners.

About a century after Hermas, the great theologian Origen (c. 185–254) wrote of the power of the name of Jesus to calm troubled minds and spirits and change hearts: "The name of Jesus can still remove distractions from the minds of men, and expel demons, and also take away diseases; and produce a marvelous meekness of spirit and complete change of character, and a humanity, and goodness, and gentleness in those individuals who do not feign themselves to be Christians."

In his book, *On the Holy Spirit,* St. Ambrose (c. 337–397), the bishop of Milan and spiritual mentor of St. Augustine, wrote that when Christ came into the world, "He spread abroad that divine Name of His throughout all creatures, not filled up by any addition (for fullness admits not of increase), but filling up the empty spaces, that His Name might be wonderful in all the world. The pouring forth, then, of His Name signifies a kind of abundant exuberance of graces and copiousness of heavenly goods, for whatever is poured forth flows over from abundance."

Meanwhile, St. Augustine (354–430) mentioned in his letter to Proba that he had received reports that the monks and hermits in the Egyptian desert "have very frequent prayers, but these are very brief." Almost certainly, one of these brief prayers was the Jesus Prayer as we know it today.

The Jesus Prayer, then, appears to have arisen from the early Christians' profound confidence in the power of the holy name of God that found its way into the monastic practice of offering brief prayers throughout the day.

The Prayer of Tenderness

The Sinai desert is a harsh, arid place, hardly an environment that conjures up tender emotions. Yet the Orthodox archimandrite Lev

Gillet (1893–1980), writing of the spirituality of the monks of St. Catherine's in the fifth century, describes their religious life as "permeated by tenderness." And what is the source of these feelings of kindheartedness? The monks' devotion to the name of Jesus. John, a monk of the sixth century who lived near Gaza in Palestine (who is best known for his friendship and correspondence with his fellow monk, St. Barsanuphius), echoed the trust the monks of Sinai had in the name of Jesus when he wrote that great saints can fight off the devil and his temptations, but "those of us who are weak can only take refuge in the name of Jesus."

During our travels Father John and I heard monks refer to "stillness," "attentiveness," and "watchfulness" as essential to silencing the passions and banishing the distractions of daily life in order to draw closer to God. "In this stillness," Hesychius of Jerusalem, also known as Hesychius the Priest (a fifth-century monk and priest) writes in the *Philokalia,* "the heart breathes and invokes, endlessly and without ceasing, only Jesus Christ who is the Son of God and Himself God." If that statement reminds you of what you have already learned of the monks' quest to say the Jesus Prayer continually, then it will not surprise you that Hesychius is the first author on record to refer explicitly to the Jesus Prayer. He says, "By persistence in the Jesus Prayer . . . the intellect, free from all images, enjoys complete quietude."

We all desire peace of heart and mind, and when Jesus soothes and refreshes a troubled heart, the man or woman who has been saved feels such joy and gratitude that he or she will never want to be separated from Christ. "None but Jesus Christ, unifier of what is disunited," Hesychius assures us, "can give your heart lasting peace from passions."

A Shift and a Revival

As I mentioned in Chapter 4, it was the monk St. Gregory of Sinai who revived the practice of the Jesus Prayer among the monasteries and hermitages of Mount Athos. It wasn't easy: when he arrived on the Holy Mountain about the year 1300 he found only three

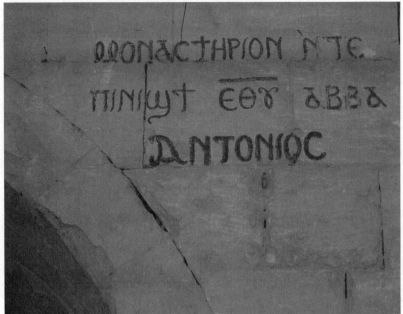

St. Antony's Monastery gate.

monks—Isaias, Cornelius, and Macarius—who practiced contemplative prayer. Nonetheless, thanks to Gregory and these three contemplative monks, the Jesus Prayer took root on Athos and from that time onward the monks of the Holy Mountain would carry the prayer throughout the Orthodox world.

Why St. Catherine's on Mount Sinai lost its influence in spreading this devotion is difficult to pin down, but it seems likely that the monastery's physical isolation played a part. By the end of the thirteenth century the Sinai Peninsula and all of the Holy Land were in Muslim hands—the last of the Crusaders having been driven out of the region in 1291. Pilgrims who wished to visit St. Catherine's, as well as monks from that monastery who wished to travel abroad to other monasteries, had to consider the risks of such a journey. If somewhere along the way they were captured by bandits or slave traders, they would never see their home again. And so the monks of St. Catherine's found themselves in many respects cut off from the Christian world.

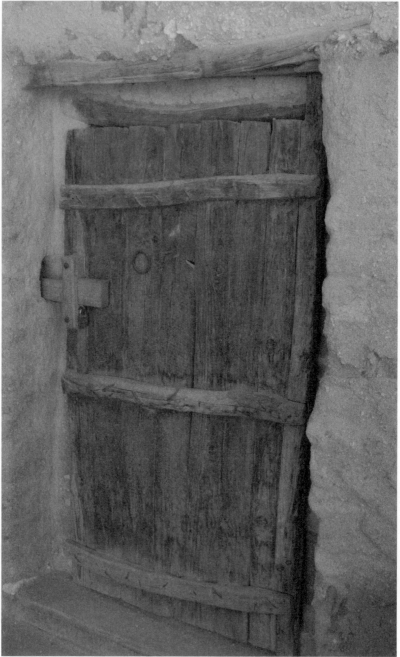

A tiny wooden door at the entrance to St. Antony Church,
St. Antony's Monastery; it is only about five feet high.

Meanwhile, on Mount Athos, St. Gregory was introducing the community to a new form of mystical prayer. We tend to regard mysticism as otherworldly, suitable for great saints but not for ordinary people. Gregory would have disputed this assumption. He regarded mystical experiences as the birthright of all Christians, a gift of the Holy Spirit bestowed at baptism but usually lying dormant until something awakens it. A desire to draw closer to God, to live a less worldly life, will awaken the mystical gift, and the practice of the Jesus Prayer will help the novice mystic along the way.

Gregory conceded that it would take practice to become adept at pushing away all distractions and focusing entirely on union with Christ. He recommended reciting the Jesus Prayer at the beginning of the day, sitting (for comfort's sake), and positioned with the head lowered so as to keep the eyes from seeking out interesting or diverting things. He advised reciting the prayer slowly, concentrating on the meaning of each word. In time, a person would be able to say with St. Paul, "It is no longer I who live, but Christ who lives in me" (Gal. 2:20).

Jesus and Mary

One of the hermits Gregory met on Athos was St. Maximus of Kapsokalyvia (died 1365). He had a wide-ranging reputation as a man who could read hearts, revealing to his visitors their deepest secrets and the sins they feared to confess. So many pilgrims made their way to distant Mount Athos and then into the wilderness to Maximus's hut that he found it necessary to retreat, time and again, deeper into the forest to regain the solitude that he sought. Each time he moved, he burned down his old hut, thus earning his surname—Kapsokalyvia, Greek for "of the burned hut." But there was no place Maximus could hide. The pilgrims always found him. For that matter, so did the messengers of the Byzantine emperors John VI Cantacuzene and John V Palaeologus, who also sought the holy man's advice.

St. Gregory visited St. Maximus, too, although since Gregory was a fellow monastic Maximus probably didn't mind. Maximus was practicing the Jesus Prayer, but he had taken it in a new direction: standing before an icon of the Holy Virgin Mary, he repeated a prayer that invoked the holy names of Jesus *and* Mary. We don't know what he said in his prayer; it was probably one of his own composition. Roman Catholics in the fourteenth century had the rosary, in which they prayed the Our Father (or Lord's Prayer) along with the Hail Mary, but the Orthodox, in spite of their intense devotion to the Theotokos, the Mother of God, had nothing comparable. What Maximus was doing was unique. Interestingly, in the seventeenth century a French Catholic priest, St. Louis de Montfort, urged the faithful to recite this brief prayer: "I am all thine and all I have is thine, O dear Jesus, through Mary, thy holy Mother."

Into the Slavic Lands

About the same time that Gregory was reviving the practice of the Jesus Prayer and Maximus was introducing a private variation on the classic formula, St. Kallistos II, patriarch of Constantinople, was writ-

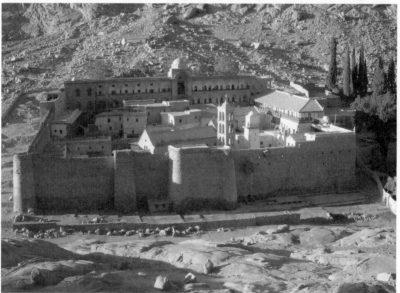

St. Catherine's Monastery from Mount Horeb.

ing a handbook for Orthodox Christians which set the Jesus Prayer at the heart of their spiritual life. Known by the peculiar name *Century,* Kallistos's book was intended for monks and nuns, but Archimandrite Lev Gillet, who immersed himself in this all-but-forgotten work in the twentieth century, believed that by making certain adaptations, any Christian could follow and profit from Kallistos's manual.

Using Kallistos's method as a starting point, the Christian who longs to deepen his or her spiritual life puts faith into action through works of mercy; reads sacred scripture daily; attends church services; receives Holy Communion worthily, with reverence and humility; at important holy days such as Easter and Christmas, keeps a nighttime vigil; and fasts on a diet of vegetables, bread, and water perhaps every Friday, the traditional day for acts of penance. All of these practices, Father Lev said, are intended to support, to reinforce the central practice: the recitation of the Jesus Prayer in order to love Jesus more deeply.

Meanwhile, from Mount Athos, the Jesus Prayer was spreading into the Slavic lands. A Russian monk on Athos, St. Nil Sorsky (1433–1508), learned how to recite this prayer; and when he returned home, he introduced it to monasteries along the Volga River. A manual for training novices at the Holy Trinity Monastery explains how to instruct them in the Jesus Prayer. It was in Ukraine and Russia that the custom arose of saying the Jesus Prayer while fingering the knots or beads of a prayer rope.

Back to the Holy Mountain

In the eighteenth century there was a monk living at Mount Athos named Nicodemus; he has become known as Nicodemus of the Holy Mountain (c. 1749–1809). While there he instructed novices in a technique that would, he believed, move the intellect into the heart.

Nicodemus's instructions to the monks were these: Every evening find a dark, quiet place where there will be no disturbance for an hour. In a comfortable seat, bow the head until the beard rests on the chest. Before beginning to pray, hold the breath briefly; then, with an inner voice, begin to recite the Jesus Prayer. Do not let the mind stray or be distracted, but keep it tuned on the words of the prayer until the prayer is the focus of mind, heart, and soul. "Set into motion the soul's will-power," Nicodemus said; "the soul must say this prayer with all its will, with all its strength, and with all its love." Of course, this was instruction to novice *monks*. While on Athos my colleagues and I—Christian laypeople—were warned by several monks and priests *not* to bow our heads and hold our breath by ourselves; this kind of use of the Jesus Prayer, they said, requires guidance from a spiritual master, and should not be done alone.

The goal of the monks and nuns who practiced—and still practice—the Jesus Prayer in this way is to move away from all that is worldly: comfort, fame, success, riches, ambition, marriage, family. A disciplined use of the Jesus Prayer makes renouncing these things easier. But what about those of us who are *in* the world, who cannot renounce our obligations? For us, the Jesus Prayer can keep us from becoming too attached to the things of the world, from making idols of our career, our salary, our car, and other status symbols. The practice of the Jesus Prayer makes it easier for us to detach ourselves from the desires and the anxieties that would distract us from deepening our spiritual life. This is what the nineteenth-century Russian bishop Theophan Govorov (1815–1894) meant when he wrote, "The essence of the practice [of the Jesus Prayer] consists in acquiring the habit of keeping the intellect on guard within the heart." This is something we can *all* aspire to, with assistance from the Jesus Prayer and by the grace of God.

The Way of the Pilgrim

In Russia in the nineteenth century, the Jesus Prayer inspired a work that has become a classic of mystical literature, *The Way of a Pilgrim*. The book itself is something of a mystery: it is written in the first person, but no one knows if it's a work of fiction or an actual autobiographical account of a wandering mystic who became a master of the Jesus Prayer. The pilgrim tells us how a starets taught him to

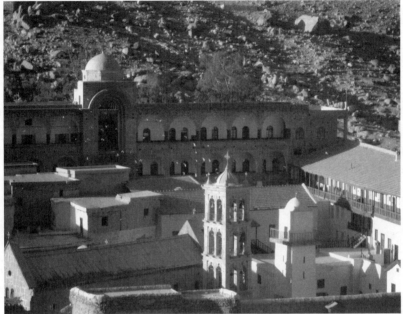

St. Catherine's Monastery from Mount Horeb, this time seen closer up.

pray the Jesus Prayer without ceasing, how it transformed his life and enabled him to endure any sorrow or suffering.

The book is at its best when the pilgrim describes what he experiences when he is praying:

> *Sometimes [when saying the Jesus Prayer] my heart would feel as if it were bursting with joy, so light was it and full of freedom and consolation. Sometimes I would feel a love toward Jesus Christ and all of God's creatures. . . . Sometimes, by invoking the name of Jesus, I was overcome with happiness, and from then on I knew the meaning of these words, "The kingdom of God is within you."*

The Jesus Prayer and *The Way of a Pilgrim* play a prominent role in J. D. Salinger's novel *Franny and Zooey*. Franny, a college student in the midst of an existential crisis, is reading *The Way of a Pilgrim* and trying to learn to pray without ceasing. Over lunch with her boyfriend she tries to explain what she's doing, but he doesn't hear her; he's caught up in his meal, the football game they will attend after lunch, the party that will follow the game. When lunch is over the boyfriend runs off to hail a taxi. Franny remains at the table, reciting the Jesus Prayer over and over. She has found the pearl of great price, while her boyfriend's mind is focused entirely on finding a cab.

Thanks in large part to *The Way of a Pilgrim,* which has been translated into many languages, the Jesus Prayer came to be known in western Europe and the United States, where a few Catholics and

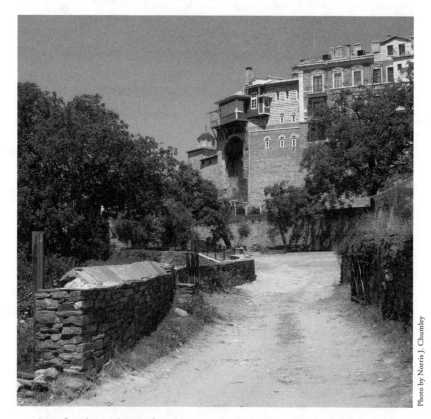

Just after the gatekeeper found our names on the list and opened the gates, we ventured forth on the dirt road leading to the great and holy Monastery of Vatopedi, on Mount Athos. Vatopedi, which means "shrubs and greenery" in Greek, is the perfect name for this thousand-year-old place of peace filled with plants and trees.

Protestants tried to practice it. The English author Evelyn Underhill (1875–1941), who had a lifelong fascination with mysticism, embraced the Jesus Prayer: "This technique [is] so simple," she wrote, "that it is within the reach of the humblest worshipper, yet so penetrating that it can introduce those who use it faithfully into the deepest mysteries of the contemplative life." Curiously, though, the Jesus Prayer is still largely unknown and not much practiced in the West. We hope that this book will help to make the prayer known and loved throughout the Western world.

Let the Prayer Do Its Work

In 1963 an Orthodox monk I mentioned earlier in this chapter, Archimandrite Lev Gillet, published what must be the finest modern work on the Jesus Prayer, entitled simply *The Jesus Prayer*. Father Lev was a Frenchman, a devout Catholic who became a Benedictine monk. He was a student of Eastern Christianity, which led to his exploration of Orthodoxy and finally to his conversion to the Orthodox Church.

Gillet numbered among his friends Catholics, Anglicans, Calvinists, Pentecostals, and Quakers, and he urged all of them to practice the Jesus Prayer. It would not be going too far to say that Father Lev made it his mission to bring the Jesus Prayer to the churches of the West.

In his book Father Lev insists that no elaborate preparations are necessary to begin the practice; just calm your restless mind, ask the Holy Spirit for help, then begin to repeat the prayer. His only warning is a simple one: do not try to force yourself to have a "mystical" experience or try to bring on a false emotionalism. Let the prayer do its work on its own. "Having begun to pronounce the name [of Jesus] with loving adoration," he writes, "all we have to do is attach ourselves to it, cling to it, and repeat it slowly, gently and quietly."

Don't rush through the repetitions of the prayer, Father Lev urges. And don't overdo it. If you become tired, stop praying. But even when you're not praying, no matter what else you may be doing, try to be

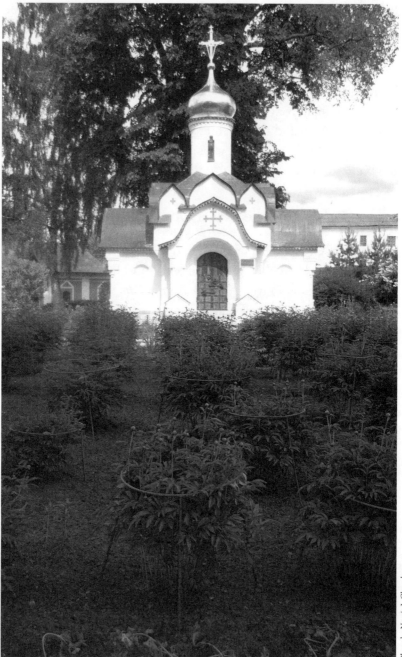

A little chapel at Sergiyev Posad Monastery in Russia, amidst a flower garden.
Perhaps a monk is inside, praying.

attentive to your desire to remain always in the presence of Jesus. The Bible describes this state as "I slept, but my heart was awake" (Song of Sol. 5:2).

What can reciting the name of Jesus do? Father Lev assures us, "The name of Jesus is a concrete and powerful means of transfiguring men into their most profound and divine reality." He urges us to say the prayer silently as we go about work, as we walk down the street, invoking the name of Jesus over everyone we see and trying always to act in a manner that will suggest to the people around us that we are trying to live for Christ.

The pilgrimage that Father John and I made, our quest to unlock the mysteries of the Jesus Prayer, was guided by all these wise and holy men and women who had experienced the spiritual, life-changing power of the prayer. Their writings about the Jesus Prayer were mystical handbooks that let us follow in the footsteps of saints.

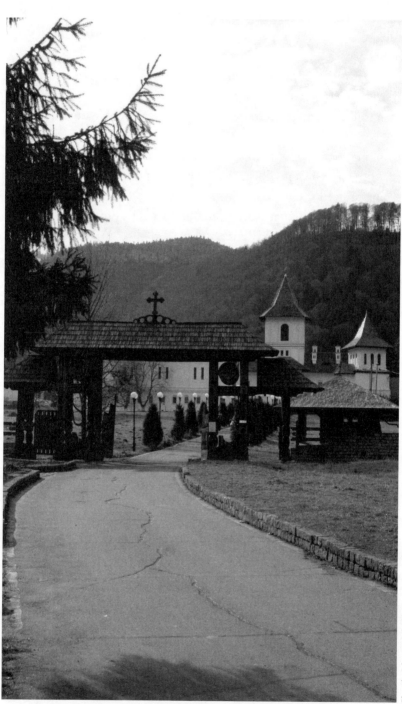

6

The Jesus Prayer
in the Painted Churches
of Romania

ROMANIA IS ALL ABOUT HOSPITALITY. I think Romanians are among the warmest, most welcoming people on earth. We were treated like royalty every second of our visit to their homeland.

I had always associated Romania with Count Dracula and with Communism (which of course is in their history), but those, I discovered, were very limited impressions. Furthermore, the fall of Communism in 1989 ended many decades of oppression: now Romania is in full bloom with its own free political independence, and Romanians are very happy people. In Romania we saw fertile farmland, thatched-roofed cottages, and two modern cities, and we experienced great warmth and abundance throughout the land.

Father John McGuckin has a wide circle of friends and colleagues there, because he was trained for and introduced to the priesthood in

---

Opposite: The road and main gate of Brâncoveanu Monastery at Sâmbăta de Sus, nestled deep in the Transylvanian mountains and woods of Romania. This is a picturesque and tranquil place of healing and spiritual renewal, with its own history of struggle and resurrection.

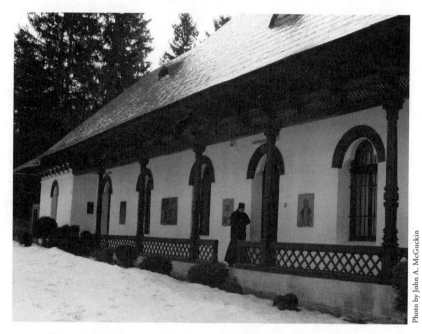

Photo by John A. McGuckin

A lone monk walks to his cell at Brâncoveanu Monastery, Sâmbăta de Sus.

Romania. Father John's Romanian connection began while he was working on his doctorate in church history. Although he's Irish and grew up in England, during the last year of his doctoral program he studied in Romania. That single year of research stretched into three years, most of it spent living at the Monastery of St. Ana, also known as Rohia, located in the northern Romanian province of Transylvania. At St. Ana he began his formation for the religious life, and was ordained a deacon there. To this day he is affectionately regarded as a special "son" of the monks and priests of St. Ana.

Brâncoveanu Monastery

We landed in Bucureşti—Bucharest—arriving late and exhausted, which was typical for this project. Father Daniel, our host in Romania, escorted us to a little town nearby, Ploeşti, where rooms had been reserved for us at the Hotel Central. Very tired but also very hungry, we dragged ourselves to the dining room, where the staff served us a magnificent Romanian feast that included stuffed cabbage, homemade sausages, potato delights, and *tuică,* an intensely potent homemade liquor, akin to vodka, distilled from plums or other end-of-season fruits. I've learned that every country has its own variety: the Italians call it *grappa,* the Greeks *ouzo,* the Turks *raki.* A little goes a long way, but I learned to enjoy a tiny shot of it.

The next morning, after fortifying ourselves with a breakfast of pierogi, more sausages, and many cups of coffee, we all climbed aboard a minibus for Brâncoveanu Monastery in Sâmbăta de Sus, a six-hour drive away. In Romania, distances are great, towns few and far between, and highways almost nonexistent. Consequently, our roundabout route on back roads took so long that we didn't arrive at Sâmbăta de Sus until late afternoon, shortly before the sun set. Nonetheless, we were greeted warmly by the abbot, who served us a variety of delicious meats and cheeses, washed down with *tuică:* in Romania, this passes for a light snack.

We wolfed down our food because we wanted to film the monastery before we lost what remained of daylight. As our film crew captured some beautiful shots of the historic monastery nestled in the Carpathian Mountains, Father John and I spoke with Father Daniel, the resident monk who had met us in Bucharest, who told us the history of the monastery. The monastery was founded late in the seventeenth century by Preda Brâncoveanu, a wealthy man, a devout son of the Romanian Orthodox Church, and the governor of the province. In 1785 an Austrian army, under the command of General Bukow, marched into Romania to annex the country for the Austro-Hungarian Empire. Brâncoveanu was one of several monasteries that Bukow ordered destroyed. The place remained in ruins until 1926; that year Metropolitan Nicolae Balan ordered the reconstruction of the monastery, which was completed and rededicated just after World War II, in 1946. Curiously, Brâncoveanu was one of the very few monasteries allowed to function during the forty-four years the country

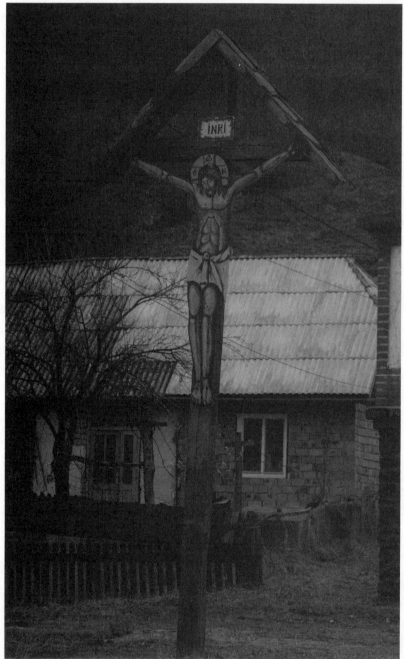

A very Romanian-style cross near the entrance of Brâncoveanu
Monastery, Sâmbăta de Sus.

was under Communist rule. Since the fall of the Communist dictator Nicolae Ceauşescu, the monastery has been renovated and expanded, with a new library for the monks and a new museum for visitors.

The Power That Thinks and the Power That Loves

One evening Father Daniel led us into one of the monastery's buildings and down a short hallway to a cell where we found a blind monk seated, reading the Bible in Braille. Father Daniel introduced us to Părintele Archimandrite Teofil Părăian, the starets of the monastery, whom I quoted in Chapter 3. "Welcome!" he said with a smile. "I am so glad you are here!" We had barely shaken hands when he began to speak fervently about the Jesus Prayer. "Wait!" I cried. "Please, Father, wait for our camera!" He laughed, nodded, and waited.

When we began again, Archimandrite Teofil corrected our terminology. We should not refer to "the Jesus Prayer," he said, because it is not a prayer *of* Jesus, but a prayer of those who call upon Jesus. "It

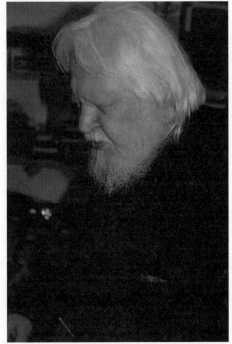

Photo by John A. McGuckin

The late starets of Brâncoveanu Monastery, Părintele Archimandrite Teofil Părăian, prays the Jesus Prayer for our salvation.

is a prayer of request," Father Teofil said, "by which we are actually asking of God whatever is necessary for the advance, for the progress of the spiritual life."

He told us he is always reminded, at the ceremony in which a monk makes his profession, that "you are worthy and you are obliged in every hour to have in your mind, in your thoughts, in your heart, and in your mouth, the name of our Lord Jesus, and to say, 'Lord Jesus Christ, Son of God, have mercy on me, a sinner.'"

Father Teofil began praying the Jesus Prayer in 1942, when he was a teenager studying to become a monk. He recalled seeing for the first time what he described as "the dirt of my own soul." It frightened him. "I couldn't imagine that in my soul one could find so much wickedness," he said. "But I also had a positive experience," he added. It was his custom, while on his way to his studies, to pray the Jesus Prayer silently. One morning he was suddenly filled with an inexpressible happiness. "I had so much joy that I felt like somebody was holding me up, and I was sure that I could not stand more joy than that. It was a gift, a precious gift, from God."

Almost every other monk and nun we met warned us not to attempt to say the Jesus Prayer incessantly without the direction of a spiritual guide, but Father Teofil was something of a rebel. He assured us that *anyone* could use it, and that God himself would never betray those who petition him in prayer.

Particularly wonderful was what Father Teofil said to us at the very end of our time with him, when I asked him what the purpose of prayer was. His response: "To make a link between prayer and mind, between mind and heart, between the power that thinks and the power that loves. So the mind that descends its awareness into the heart is not an activity of the human being, it is a work of God. What we are doing is that we pray to God for the unity of our own being, the whole being."

I recently heard that Archimandrite Teofil had "fallen asleep in the Lord," as the monks say. He died on October 29, 2009. I was sad to hear this, but happy that now he will be with his Creator.

The Breath of the Heart

The morning after our conversation with Father Teofil I awoke very early, around 5:30 A.M., to find two members of our group, Pat Gallo and Dwight Grimm, already set up with cameras, filming the sunrise against the lovely sculpted wooden columns that stood outside the rows of the monks' cells.

On this day we would be driving to a monastery that had special significance for Father John: he was ordained a deacon there. We were traveling in the thick of winter, and the roads were slick with ice, so it took many hours to cover the 300 miles from Brâncoveanu to St. Ana's Monastery in Rohia, but it proved to be a marvelous drive through the remote land of the snowcapped Carpathian Mountains. We shared the road with horse-drawn carts driven by predominantly elderly Romanian farm couples. We passed old farmsteads with chickens in the yard, cows grazing for scarce tufts of grass in the pastures, and barns piled high with bales of hay that had been hand-gathered and carted in from the frozen fields. This felt more than rural—it was as if we had stepped back in time.

At last we arrived at a little village tucked in the crevices of the mountain range, in the middle of the deepest forests of Transylvania. In the center of the village stood a wooden gateway painted white and bearing an icon of Christ at the center of the arch. A little hand-painted sign read, "St. Ana's Monastery." As we traveled up the drive we saw a collection of old chapels and churches, along with newly built cells for the monks, a refectory for meals, and a lovely guest-house, all embellished with beautiful wood carvings.

Father John was greeted like a returning rock star. Although it had been fifteen years since he lived at Rohia, all the monks turned out to welcome him home.

Because it was late afternoon with the sun about to set, the monks could not dawdle to chat with us after that hearty welcome, but had to hurry to vespers. We unpacked our cameras and followed them through a maze of corridors to a tiny underground chapel, its walls

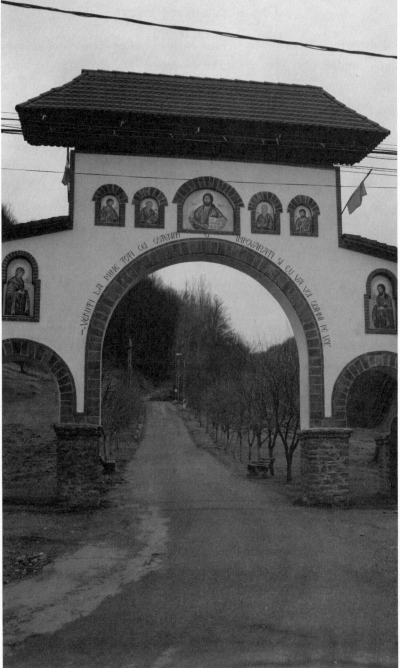

The welcoming front gate of St. Ana's Monastery at Rohia in Romania.

covered with icons, the air thick with incense as the monks chanted heavenly chords in Romanian harmony. Carrying one of the cameras, I flicked off my shoes and wandered around filming. Right up to the altar I went; right through the monks, singing and chanting (they gave me most curious looks); past icons with glowing eyes; round the corners of carved antiquities.

One particular chanting monk watched us intently as we filmed. After the service, I learned he was His Eminence Iustin Sigheteanul, a bishop and the abbot of Rohia Monastery. He had been expecting us and very kindly granted us an interview after the evening service.

He began by explaining that the underground chapel the community was using was temporary; they were building an entirely new church, to be completed in another year or so. The original church, built in 1926, was "modest," he said, and during the oppressive years of Communist rule when only one monk was permitted to live at Rohia, it was forbidden to make any repairs or upgrades. By 1989, the year the Romanians overthrew the Ceauşescu regime, the Rohia church was in dilapidated condition. Since the revival of the Romanian Orthodox Church and of monastic life in general, the monks at Rohia have been able to build a fine new church. There is a fresh air of renewal at Rohia, a certain vibrancy and energy that is contagious. We felt it not only at the monastery, but everywhere we traveled in Romania. Thanks to countless vampire movies inspired by Bram Stoker's nineteenth-century novel *Dracula,* there is a general misperception that Romania is a creepy place. Nothing could be farther from the truth: as I noted earlier, the countryside is glorious; the people are warm, generous, and hospitable; and in monasteries and convents across the land, the mystical tradition long suppressed under Ceauşescu has been revived.

During our stay at Rohia we were invited to the new library to meet the former starets, Archimandrite Serafim Man. He was a gracious, energetic man, despite suffering from a serious illness. I'll never forget how he talked about prayer. "One of the greatest gifts which God has given to us is the possibility to be in permanent contact [with him] at any time, at any place," Father Serafim said. "Prayer is the breath of the heart. It is the mouth of heaven, of paradise. It is the mouth of the angels. When we pray, we are actually similar to the angels, who are in a state of ceaseless praise for God. Therefore, we are told that prayer should be ceaseless."

He was elderly and frail, his voice barely rising above a whisper, yet the love and grace of God shone brightly in him.

The Church in Romania

Two thousand years ago Romania, as the name suggests, was a province of the Roman Empire. In fact, it was the easternmost imperial province in Europe, and although remote from Rome, it was important to the empire: it gave the Romans access to the Black Sea and the great mercantile cities along its shores.

Tradition claims that the apostle St. Andrew, the brother of St. Peter, established the Christian Church in Romania, but in fact no one knows when Christianity arrived in Romania, nor who introduced it. We *do* know that there were Christians in the Roman legions and in the imperial administration; perhaps it was one of these soldiers or bureaucrats who planted the faith in Romania. From archaeological evidence we know that there were Christians in the country by the year 150 and that many Romanian Christians were martyred during the persecution of Christianity under Emperor Decius in 249 and under Emperor Diocletian in 304. Yet as was true throughout the empire, the new faith flourished in spite of persecution. By 311, Romanian Christians were served by fourteen bishops. Soon thereafter the first monastic communities were founded in the region of Dobrogea along the Black Sea.

Because the developing Christian Church in Romania was geographically closer to Constantinople than to Rome, it adopted the Byzantine liturgy that is common to all branches of the Orthodox and Eastern Rite Catholic Churches. It would eventually be known as the Romanian Orthodox Church.

During the centuries when Romania was occupied by the Ottoman Turks and then by the Austro-Hungarian Empire, the Romanian

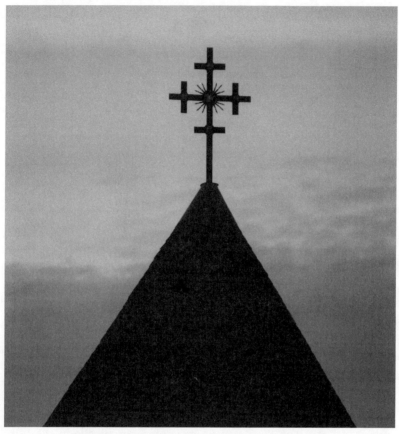

Photo by John A. McGuckin

A Romanian cross at the top of a chapel in Transylvania.

Church was the spiritual and cultural touchstone of the people. Consequently, when the Communists seized power in 1947, the Romanian Church came under severe attack. Three archbishops were murdered; thirteen bishops were arrested. Two thousand monks were driven from their monasteries, and 1,500 priests and laypeople were imprisoned. The church's 2,300 elementary schools were closed, as were fifteen of eighteen seminaries, all twenty-four of its high schools, and half of its monasteries. Those monasteries that were permitted to remain open were staffed by a tiny handful of monks—in some places by a solitary monk (including Rohia, as noted above). The persecution lasted into the 1980s, when the Ceauşescu government demolished two dozen architecturally and historically significant churches in Bucharest and announced plans to destroy churches in the rural villages as well.

Since the fall of the Communist regime in 1989, the Romanian Orthodox Church has seen a tremendous revival. Nearly 87 percent of the population identify themselves as Romanian Orthodox. More than 8,000 monks and nuns live in the country's 637 monasteries and convents. The Romanian Orthodox Church has reopened its schools and seminaries and has founded new institutions, such as clinics and soup kitchens, as well as facilities to shelter children and the elderly and to help victims of domestic violence, drug addicts, and people infected with HIV/AIDS.

"This Is the Mystery"

We were all up very early again the next morning for a long, long drive to the city of Baia Mare, where we were scheduled to interview His Eminence Archbishop Justinian Chira Maramureşeanul, the highest-ranking church official in the region of Maramureş.

The archbishop welcomed us to his residence and had some special words of welcome for Father John. "Brother John," he said, "we have been waiting for you for a long time, because I know you have a very important task. You have a mission: you are an apostle in the New World and in the Western world in general, which knows too little, I'm afraid, about the Eastern world."

Prompted by our questions, Archbishop Justinian then spoke about prayer. "We have three virtues: fasting, almsgiving, and prayer," he said. "This is mentioned in the Gospel according to Matthew, chapter 6. But out of those, prayer is the key. It is a means of gaining direct contact with God. . . . [W]e can say prayer is the virtue of virtues.

He continued: "In the liturgical life of [the Romanian Orthodox] Church there is a very important hymn that says, 'Let us leave aside every human concern.' When you reach into yourself and you get rid of any kind of human concern, you are focusing all of your spiritual and intellectual powers; you are aware that you don't speak in vain but you speak to a Person who is love, [and] you become aware that

God is present. I don't see him when I pray, but I know him. I understand he is listening to my prayer. This is what the people today should learn, because people have forgotten how to pray.

"So if a novice should ask me to teach him the Jesus Prayer, I would say, 'Start with the first step; say, "Jesus Christ, Son of God, have mercy upon me," and say it without ceasing when you go to work or to the office or when you drive. Say this until it becomes a habit. Then stop saying it and start doing it silently only in your thoughts.' The thought itself becomes a prayer, saying, 'Jesus Christ, Son of God, have mercy upon me.' All alien thoughts are set aside. The mind is no longer concerned with the daily occupations. Now you start having the pure thoughts, and pure thoughts exercise a tendency toward the heart and it starts changing the heart.

"This is the mystery," Archbishop Justinian concluded. "This is the sacrament."

The archbishop said all this in rapid-fire Romanian, and although I couldn't understand a word (until his response was later translated for me), I tried to intuit what he was saying. Perhaps he recognized my intention, because he suddenly reached out and took my hand with his, and he put his other hand on my chest. Immediately I felt a truly strong presence of God coursing through me. Deeply moved, I began to cry.

Sister Irina

I had barely recovered from the interview with Archbishop Justinian when it was time to leave, because we had an appointment with an abbess. Up to this point, we had been unable to convince any nuns to appear in the film. In Egypt and Greece, at convent after convent, abbess after abbess turned us down. But not in Romania! We were on our way to Voroneț Monastery in Gura Humorului, Moldavia, called by some the "Sistine Chapel of the East" because of the magnificent mural painted on the exterior walls of its church—where, despite the elements, the painting remains in magnificent condition. Dating from 1547, the fresco depicts scenes from the Last Judgment.

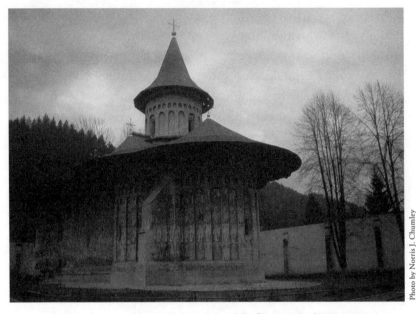

Photo by Norris J. Chumley

Perhaps the most famous "painted church" of Romania: the Voroneț
Monastery church located near the town of Gura Humorului, Moldavia.

It is famous in the art world for its unique shade of deep cerulean,
known as "Voroneț Blue."

Abbess Sister Irina Pântescu met us at our scheduled time and was
clearly delighted to talk with us and participate in the film. She began
by speaking of her calling to the religious life and stated plainly that
she didn't see women playing a role much different (or lesser, as some
believe) in the Romanian Church. Yes, male priests conduct the services and offer the Eucharist, she conceded, but the sisters are also very
involved. "Everyone prays together," she explained. "The occupations
of monks and nuns are the same." And that occupation, of course, is
prayer. All nuns and all monks pray for the world, all the time.

As we chatted, Sister Irina gave us a grand tour, the highlight being
the Church of St. George, which, we discovered is as splendidly fres-
coed inside as it is outside. It was built in 1488 by Prince Stephen the
Great of Moldava in thanksgiving for his victory over the Ottoman
Turks. During our tour we met some of the sisters, who were explaining the interior frescoes and icons to groups of visitors.

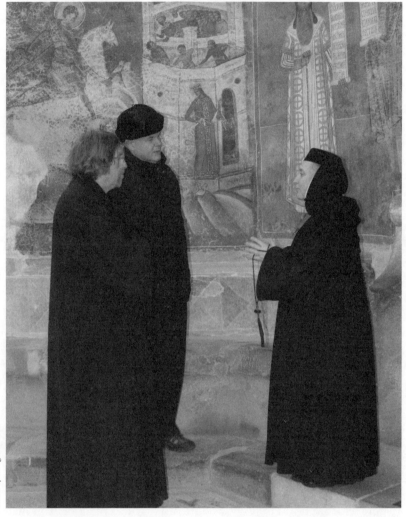

Photo by Dwight Grimm

Sister Johana narrates the story of the Last Judgment on the west wall of the Voroneţ Monastery church for Father John and Norris Chumley. Note the "sword" prayer rope around her arm; she uses it to continually pray the Jesus Prayer.

Just before we left, Sister Irina demonstrated how she prays the Jesus Prayer as a prayer walk. I had never seen such a thing. In fact, none of the monks and bishops we had spoken with had even hinted that the Jesus Prayer could be practiced this way. It is strikingly simple. Every two steps she said a phrase of the prayer quietly under her

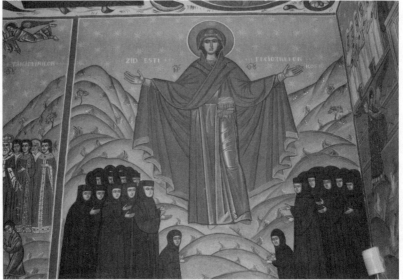

A wall mural icon of the Holy Mother of God in the recesses of the confessional room at Voroneț Monastery chapel. She guides all the sisters, below.

breath. The first two steps, "Lord Jesus Christ." The next two steps, "Son of God." Another two steps, "Have mercy on me." Step, step, "A sinner."

While Sister Irina never explained why she finds this to be a helpful practice, I know from my studies that linking breathing to the Jesus Prayer originated on Mount Athos in the fourteenth century with St. Gregory Palamas. That method, mentioned in Chapter 4, links the prayer from mind to body, as does Sister Irina's practice. You may find one of their variations helpful.

A Child in Her Parents' Arms

A short distance from Voroneț is one of the largest convents in the world, Văratec Monastery, the home to approximately 600 nuns. The term "convent" is one I use because many readers are probably familiar with it; the nuns say "monastery." The abbess, Sister Josephina Giosanu, was awaiting our arrival. A youthful woman, Sister

Josephina spent many hours with us. She gave us interviews and a tour, of course, but she also introduced us to the convent's neighbors, and permitted us to take our cameras into her cell and into that of her aunt, who is also a nun at Văratec. This was a very special privilege. Because monks and nuns have left the world and don't really want the world to follow them, it's a unique experience to be able to glimpse an ascetic's private life. I believe that we were given these gifts because these sisters care about us—much more than we realize.

Sister Josephina talked a lot about young people and those who are living in the world. She recalled that when she was a teenager she longed for a life of peace. Through prayer, she felt called by God to seek out nuns and monks. The conversations she had with these monastics led her to the decision to enter the convent. She was invited into the monastery at Văratec when she was in her teens and has lived there for thirty years.

Most monasteries welcome pilgrims—seekers of God—for brief visits only, and only to the public churches. Many monks confided to me, sadly, that many of these visitors disturb their silence and their practice of prayer and contemplation. Văratec seemed different: there were many townspeople freely entering and exiting the convent grounds unescorted, and many of the nuns were speaking with these visitors. Sister Josephina not only gave us a great deal of her time but also paused as we walked through the convent grounds to chat with children and their parents who were also visiting Văratec at the time.

This set Văratec apart from the other sacred sites we had visited, but to Sister Josephina there was nothing exceptional in her conduct or that of her nuns. She explained that there are nuns who find it their vocation to be with the pilgrims, and that to do so is their "obedience," the sacrifice or offering they make for the good of the convent and for the good of the souls of the people they meet. Other sisters are happiest in solitary occupations such as sewing, weaving, and painting icons, while still others (including many of the nuns at Văratec) keep to themselves, living in silence and prayer, offering their prayers to God for the salvation of the world.

Văratec is very large, comprising seventy acres with 180 houses and other buildings, as well as three churches that are in operation throughout the day and night. The name Văratec means "like summer" or "mild climate," and we felt this difference in the weather when we were there. Although it was the middle of winter, Văratec's microclimate was milder than we had experienced elsewhere.

Sister Josephina told us that after the fall of the Communist government in 1989, there were many, many young women who came and asked to join the community. Most did not stay very long, for a host of reasons. The monastic life is not an easy one, but for those who embrace this particular way of life, there are tremendous consolations. Something Sister Josephina said about living only for God as a nun has really stayed with me: "A child keeps quiet when she feels the arms of her parents and feels the joy of being with her parents. And I think it is the same feeling when a novice comes and when she finds silence. When she finds herself in such an environment she feels the love of God, and she feels that joy which that little child would in the parents' arms."

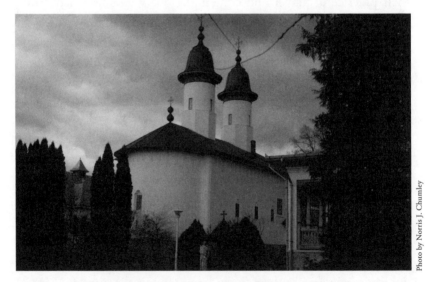

The main church, one of five at Văratec Monastery, a recently
settled convent in northeastern Romania.

"The Spirit Blows Where He Wishes"

In the mountains of Moldavia we found Agapia Monastery, named after a forest-dwelling hermit. "Agapia," by the way, comes from the Greek term for "spiritual love." We were met at the door of the church by Mother Maria Balan, an English-speaking nun who invited us inside to see some sublime icons, painted by Nicolae Grigorescu in the nineteenth century.

During our conversation with Mother Maria, she discussed the important role of women in the Orthodox Church, and also what it means to a nun to be "married" to Christ. She would not, however, tell us, as she put it, of "the delightedness of meeting with the bridegroom." I left that subject alone, of course. It must be truly heavenly to be married to God, though, judging by the joy reflected in her eyes and the glee in her smile.

On prayer she explained, "The peace of the heart is something ineffable you can't speak of. It is a gift of God, the grace of the Holy Spirit. And the Spirit blows where he wishes."

At one point our conversation turned to the subject of sin and forgiveness. I admitted to Mother Maria that in my life I had made many mistakes and had sinned repeatedly, but I had asked God for help. "We're *all* sinners, dear Norris," she said, and gave me a little bottle of holy water. I have it to this day, kept in a special place in our home.

In the convent's church we joined Mother Maria in prayer, after which she took us to meet Ioan Mihoc, a nun and professor who is the director of the St. John of Hozeva Lay Academy for Women, housed in a separate building on Agapia grounds. In a classroom at the academy we were treated to an angelic performance of several prayers sung by a choir of young women students.

We were reluctant to leave Agapia—the remote mountain setting is enchanting and Mother Maria is a wise and gentle teacher of the spiritual life—but we had an appointment the next morning in Iaşi with the highest bishop in the land.

The Uncreated Light

The metropolitan's palace in Iaşi is a grand old building filled with elaborately decorated chapels and churches; even the offices and meeting rooms are embellished with gilded woodwork and lovely murals. Before he was elevated to the episcopate, His Eminence Metropolitan Daniel Ciobotea was a professor of theology who specialized in the theology of icons. During our meeting the conversation turned naturally to icons, and Bishop Daniel—who speaks English fluently—said something that surprised me. "We don't need to use images during prayer," he said. It was a statement that took us all aback, given that icons are everywhere in the Orthodox world. "True prayer," Bishop Daniel explained, "is prayer without imagination, without forms, without images." Then, as if he anticipated my next question, he added, "And at the same time, the Orthodox churches and especially monasteries have plenty of icons."

He showed us several icons in the palace chapel. "What is important in the icon," he said, "is not only the face of Christ or of the Virgin Mary, or of the saints, but the light beyond the face, which is the light eternal, the uncreated light. The glory of God in which we are called to share—that is the purpose of true prayer. In fact, the icon is a guide to the eternal light of God. It means the beauty of his presence, his communion. So the foretaste of the eternal light of God, of the glory of God, of the beauty of God, of the love of God, is in the experience." This was the most beautiful, most profound, and most perfectly articulated explanation of icons I'd ever heard.

From our discussion of the mystical significance of icons, we segued into a question about laypeople praying the Jesus Prayer. "It's not necessary to live in the desert to be isolated from the world," the metropolitan said. "What is important is to be united with God. Even in New York City, or in Bucharest, or in Iaşi, or in the village, the stress from outside or from the society is pressing us to find alternatives, to find a new way, the interior way, in order to approach and to change the world."

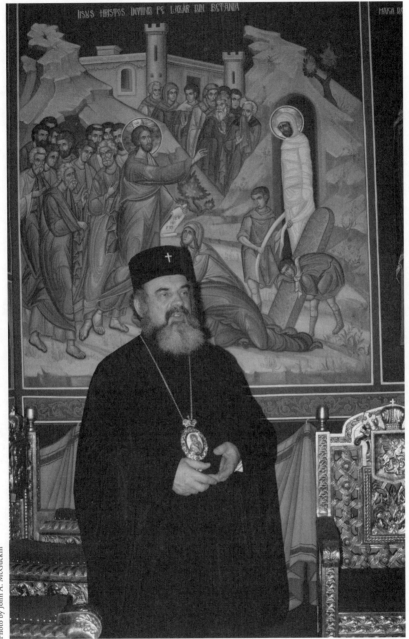

Photo by John A. McGuckin

His Beatitude Dr. Daniel Ciobotea, now patriarch of Romania,
when he was Metropolitan of Moldavia.

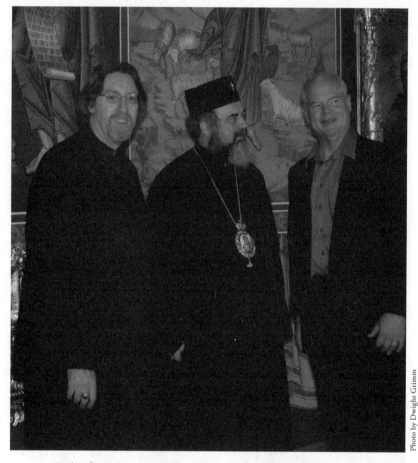

Photo by Dwight Grimm

Right after our interview, His Beatitude Dr. Daniel Ciobotea, now patriarch of Romania, showed Father John and Norris Chumley the beautiful chapel of the metropolitan's palace.

At midday the metropolitan invited us to join him for lunch; it was the traditional Romanian banquet to which by now we had become happily accustomed. His Eminence had me sit right next to him, as somehow we had immediately bonded. He had read my book *The Joy of Weight Loss* and was himself finishing writing a book on food. We encouraged each other to try only small bites of the myriad dishes, eating slowly, praying together with every bite for God's grace to not overeat—a powerful temptation to resist at such a glorious meal.

The Patriarch

Next we had appointment to meet the senior-most Romanian Orthodox church official: His Beatitude Patriarch Theoctist. I was embarrassed to have nothing to wear but rumpled clothes for this important meeting. I wrote in my journal, "Nothing like wearing dirty clothes for an audience with the pope!" But I had no choice: our work and travel schedule had been so demanding that there had been absolutely no time whatsoever to go to a laundry, and since we rarely stayed long in any place, we couldn't even send our clothes out to be cleaned.

It was a short drive from Iaşi to Bucharest, to the patriarch's residence. We were waiting for him in a large conference room, as instructed, when at last the door opened and a small white-haired man in glowing white robes and a bejeweled patriarch's miter entered, followed by his entourage of about a half-dozen clerics. He was hunched over and had trouble walking, but when he looked at us I saw a lovely warm and glowing expression in his eyes.

Father John had coached me the previous evening on the proper protocol when meeting a patriarch, so I knelt down and reached for his hand to kiss it. There are some high church officials who, upon meeting a visitor, instantly hold out their hand to be kissed, and others who, perhaps out of humility, don't *assume* that the kiss is coming. Patriarch Theoctist was definitely one of the latter.

He sat down, and we were formally introduced by one of his lieutenants, who mentioned to His Beatitude that Father John and I were from New York. Instantly the patriarch began to regale us—in Romanian—with memories of his trips to the United States, and especially of New York, which he has visited seven times. Through the translator he described New York City as a "very famous suburb," and recalled going to "shops where they want you to buy something, but they didn't care about the profit." Apparently the storekeepers had let the patriarch shop at wholesale prices, or had given him some gifts. He must have visited the Cathedral of St. John the Divine in New York City, as he remembered a "cathedral under construction that is taking many years to finish." He'd been briefed on "Romania's spiritual son," Father John, and was happy that he had come back "home" to visit. It was all delightful.

The whole tone of our meeting changed when His Beatitude began to speak most sincerely and eloquently about prayer. "Man has a very powerful will—so powerful that even God himself does not break it," he explained. "And by this [God] is actually showing that man is in the likeness of God. Without man's will he could not make any progress on the way to goodness. So out of all the gifts that God grants the human being, we believe that freedom is one of the most important."

The subject of freedom is an important one in Romania, since for many years of Communist rule the Romanians had none. As noted earlier, since the fall of the Communist regime just over twenty years ago Romania has begun to rebuild and restore many beautiful and important buildings and churches that the Ceaușescu government damaged or left to deteriorate.

When he spoke of prayer, His Beatitude likened it to "dinner with God." It is an apt metaphor, especially given the importance Romanians place on meals and hospitality. He went on to say that when we pray, it is in "a common voice." That blended prayer can create a true fellowship, especially when people from varied traditions, beliefs, and perspectives pray together. "Prayer is so powerful that it reduces any distance between us and God so we can see him, can approach him very easily through prayer."

He went on to tell us a story about a young believer who insisted that he saw no use—no benefits or results—from his earnest efforts to pray; the boy felt that God simply didn't hear his prayers. A spiritual elder instructed the boy to get a basket, take it to the river, and fill it with water. He tried to comply, but every time he lifted the basket from the river, the water leaked out. Angry and frustrated, he returned to the elder with a waterlogged but empty basket. The task, he told the elder, had been pointless. Not true, the elder replied. By immersing the basket in the river multiple times it had been cleansed multiple times. What the river water did to the basket, prayer does to the soul. This was a lesson in receiving grace from God in ways we don't always realize—in ways of purification we don't know are needed.

At one point in our interview I felt so comfortable with the patriarch that I was able to gather up the courage to ask a question that had been in my mind for a while. "Is there a devil?" I asked hesitantly. "Is the devil, or evil, real?"

I asked this question for a couple of reasons, beyond my own personal religious searching. First, we had encountered many images of the devil in Romania—a great deal more than in other locations. There was a carving of the devil near the entrance to the patriarchal residence, for example, and depictions of the devil in icons in the patriarchal chapel. Second, many monks and nuns had explained that there is more to their lives than peace and tranquillity; there is also struggle—to resist temptation, to resist evil. That is part of the appeal of the Jesus Prayer, they said: it restores peace to people's lives, and it does so by directing penitents onto the path of righteousness, which leads to God. I wanted to delve a little deeper into what that struggle was about, so I took a chance and asked the patriarch about the devil.

Again, my fears about his potential inapproachability were unjustified. His Beatitude replied, "The devil is so real, he is right in this room with us!" There was silence all around as we waited for the patriarch to elucidate this startling statement.

"There is always, everywhere, a force that is trying to disturb our peace," the patriarch said, "trying to undermine our efforts, derailing us from communion with God." That force is the devil.

Only a short time after we arrived back in the United States, we heard the news that His Beatitude Patriarch Theoctist had "fallen asleep in the Lord." Our friend Metropolitan Daniel was chosen to succeed Theoctist as patriarch. It's more than likely that our filmed interview with Patriarch Theoctist was his last.

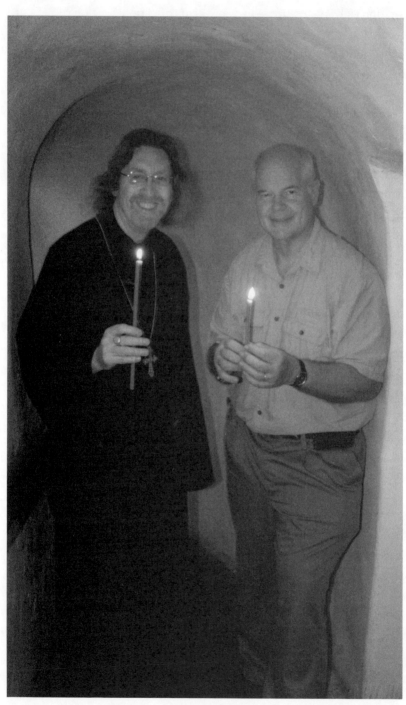

7

Following the Jesus Prayer
into the Caves of Kiev

T HE FIRST PERSON WE MET when we arrived at the Kiev airport was Igor Issayev, the guide who had been selected for us
by Bohdan Movchan, a consul at Ukraine's Embassy to the United
Nations in New York. Our friend Bohdan could not have made a
better choice: Igor, who works with the American Business Center in
Ukraine, proved to be a highly knowledgeable guide to Kiev. Greet-
ing us as if we were old friends, he told us there were not many films
being made in Kiev, especially not of monasteries.

We had come to Kiev for one reason—to visit the world-renowned
Pecherskaya Lavra, also known as the Monastery of the Caves
(*perchera* is the Ukrainian word for "cave"). A monk from Mount
Athos in Greece, known today as St. Antony of the Caves (c. 983–
1073), founded the monastery in 1051, not long after the prince of Kiev,
St. Vladimir (956–1015), converted to Christianity. The Pecherskaya
Lavra rises up a series of terraces on a steep slope above the Dnieper

---

Opposite: Father John and Norris Chumley invite you into the caves under
the Pecherskaya Lavra (Monastery of the Caves), in Kiev, Ukraine. You will
need a candle, as it is very dark!

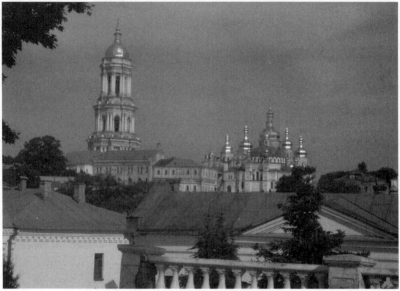

Photo by Dwight Grimm

The Great Lavra Bell Tower and St. Sophia Cathedral at the Pecherskaya
Lavra in Kiev, Ukraine. A UNESCO World Heritage Site, the tower and
church are neither owned nor operated by the monks; they are run by the state,
via its National Kiev-Pechersk Historic-Cultural Preserve, and are now
museums. There are several churches and chapels that were returned to the
monastery, however, after the fall of the Soviet government.

River. There are several sections, each with its own massive defensive
masonry wall. The city of Kiev lies all around the monastery, yet the
Pecherskaya Lavra, screened by thick woods and shielded by its walls,
seems set apart from the busy capital of Ukraine.

For almost 900 years the Pecherskaya Lavra was a nursery of saints
and a center of Orthodox spirituality and scholarship. As an example of the latter, the first printing press in Kiev was established at
the monastery in 1615. During the first years of the twentieth century, approximately 1,200 monks and novices lived at the monastery.
After the Revolution of 1917, Soviet authorities confiscated many of
the monastery's sacred treasures, mistreated the relics of the saints in
the caves, and converted the Pecherskaya Lavra into a museum. The
monks were imprisoned, sent to labor camps, or shot.

Photo by John A. McGuckin

Under the eaves of Dormition Cathedral at the Pecherskaya Lavra in Kiev.

After World War II, Joseph Stalin permitted a portion of the Pecherskaya Lavra to reopen as a Russian—not Ukrainian—Orthodox monastery. The Pecherskaya Lavra was not returned to the Ukrainian Orthodox Church until 1992, one year after the collapse of the Soviet Union.

The monastery is rich in splendid architecture—particularly the main church, Dormition Cathedral, built of white stone in the Baroque style and crowned with golden onion domes. Tragically, the original church was destroyed in 1941 during the Nazi invasion of Ukraine. It has been rebuilt, but it is not owned or operated by the Ukrainian Orthodox Church; it belongs to the Ukrainian government, which runs it as a museum. The cathedral, which is now a UNESCO World Heritage Site, was off-limits to our cameras, but we had free access to all the other churches and chapels within the monastery, as well as to the famous caves.

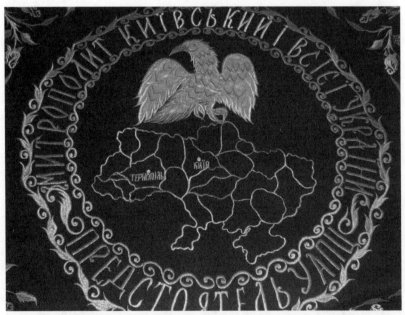

This is a special rug for bishops and high-ranking church officials to stand on during liturgical services. It depicts ancient Ukraine and old Russia. From the Pecherskaya Lavra, Kiev, Ukraine.

Father Cyril Hovorun, the head of the Ukrainian Orthodox Church's Office of External Affairs, was our host. Having been trained and educated in England, where he received a doctorate, Father Cyril spoke perfect English. Given his high position in the administration of the Ukrainian Orthodox Church, he proved invaluable in gaining for us extensive access to the holy places inside the monastery, as well as persuading members of the monastic community to speak with us on-camera.

Although we arrived late in the day, several hours after the monks' dinner hour, Father Cyril was waiting for us at the monastery guesthouse. He welcomed us warmly and suggested a bistro near the monastery's main gate where we could have dinner. We were still operating on foreign time and not very sleepy, so after our meal we went out to get some footage of the monastery grounds at night. The moon was aglow, illuminating the old stone walls and reflecting off the golden onion domes. Several times we encountered monks softly chanting prayers to God as they walked along. I wanted to stop and make conversation, but it didn't feel right. I tried sending a smile their way, but they didn't even look up. They were completely absorbed in their union with God.

The Caves

We held our first interview the next morning with Father Cyril. An articulate man, he was particularly helpful in setting the scene, providing a brief history of the Pecherskaya Lavra. "The core of what we call Russian Orthodoxy—Russian tradition and Orthodoxy—has spread out to all points of the globe, including western Europe, both Americas, Japan, and Australia," he said, sounding professorial. "That tradition started from this exact place, because this was the place where the people of Rus, ancient Rus, the people of Kiev, were baptized by St. Vladimir, the Apostle of the Lands of Rus. And this monastery became a point where people who were baptized some years before got access to the spiritual treasures, the monastic treasures of Orthodoxy."

Father Cyril told us that the founder of the monastery, St. Antony, had learned the ways of silent prayer—*hesychasm*—and contemplation on Mount Athos in Greece. When he returned to Kiev, he lived as a hermit in a cave above the banks of the Dnieper River. His devotion was such that he attracted disciples who inhabited other caves, until gradually a community began to form. It was a cenobitic community, or a group of monks who shared meals and occasionally prayed together, though they still lived separately. As St. Antony's community grew, some of his monks traveled abroad, founding new monasteries. In time, Father Cyril explained, these new monasteries sent out "missionaries who went as far as to the lands of Siberia, [where they] evangelized the pagans who lived there."

I was eager to begin filming, and Father Cyril had found the perfect assistants to help us with that—a young newlywed couple, Anthony and Helen Vovchenko. Anthony had graduated recently from the monastery's theological seminary and was training to be a parish priest. Helen, who would serve as our translator, was the daughter and granddaughter of priests. The couple had married only one month earlier and were so in love it was delightful to be with them.

Our first request was to film in the caves beneath the Pecherskaya Lavra. To our delight, Anthony and Helen made all the necessary arrangements within a few hours. Unlike the pilgrims who stood in extremely long lines to enter the caves, we were given full access after the caves had closed for the day.

After the last of the pilgrims had gone, Anthony and Helen led us inside a small chapel. From there, a doorway opened onto a long flight of stairs that led down about fifty vertical feet. From there, the entryway, we were greeted by a hermit who escorted us into a network of tunnels. Along the tunnels were small caves or cells, once the dwelling places of monks, today the shrines of countless saints. In most cases the bones were wrapped in shrouds and laid out in caskets with no lids so that the faithful could see the remains of the saints. We saw the relics of St. Ilya Muromets, a legendary thirteenth-century knight who defended Kiev and the surrounding region from the Mongols, and of St. Vladimir Bogoyavlensky, a metropolitan of Kiev who was murdered by Bolsheviks early in the twentieth century.

The tunnels are completely plastered over and painted white, with electric lights dispelling the gloom. The walls are decorated with murals and icons, some of them centuries old, hung on spots that were unplastered. Amid the tombs and tunnels are two underground places of worship, the Church of the Nativity of Christ, where novices for centuries have been tonsured (a rite that symbolizes the beginning of their monastic life), and the Church of the Annunciation, a grotto with primitive stone chairs and an ancient altar.

I mentioned earlier the unusual smell we had encountered in the ossuary at St. Catherine's. That smell is one of the things that struck me the most here in the caves. As I noted earlier, the skulls of saints occasionally give off myrrh, an intensely fragrant oil that pilgrims believe has miraculous healing powers. Only certain skulls beneath the Pecherskaya Lavra give off the scent for only a few weeks or days in the year, and it's unpredictable when it will appear. We experienced the great grace to be filming in the catacombs when one skull was exuding myrrh. It was a scent unlike anything I had ever encountered before: a mixture of citrus and herb, sweet and sour, with a touch of an alkaline, chalky aroma. My words don't come close to describing this perfume. Honestly, it's a little strange smelling an ancient skull, but I'm so glad to have had the opportunity; it's an experience like none I've ever had before, nor am I likely ever to have it again!

During our exploration of the caves we encountered the *kellia,* or cells, of unique monks, called *anchorites,* who practiced the strictest form of enclosure. Monks who felt called to live as total recluses were sealed inside their cells with stones and mortar, with only a hole four inches wide and five inches high through which bread and water could be passed. These ascetics lived in complete darkness, passing their lives in constant prayer. At their death their bodies were left inside their cells, undisturbed, where they still lie to this day.

We were in the caves for hours and hours. Some ascetics a century ago claimed that the tunnels in the caves were so long that they reached all the way to Moscow. That's an exaggeration, of course, but the tunnels are very long indeed. I'd never experienced claustrophobia before, but I began to in these caves, and I was very happy when at last we returned to ground level.

Equal to the Apostles

Father Cyril was correct when he said that it was from Kiev that Christianity had spread across Ukraine and Russia, and it was introduced by two very unlikely missionaries.

In 945 Igor, prince of Kiev, led an army against the Drevlians, a neighboring tribe and vassal state that had rebelled and refused to pay its annual tribute. At the sight of Igor's army, the Drevlian prince backed down and paid up. Igor was leading his troops home when it occurred to him that he should have collected a penalty payment from the Drevlians. With only a small retinue, he turned back. The Drevlian prince listened to Igor's demand, but instead of handing over more gold, he had Igor and his small band of followers killed.

When word of the murder reached Igor's widow, Olga, she didn't take it well. To avenge her husband she had some Drevlians buried alive, some burned in a sauna, and others massacred as they sat at a banquet; finally, she destroyed the Drevlian capital, selling all survivors into slavery.

After ruling Kiev and the surrounding region for nine years, Olga traveled south to Constantinople to forge an alliance with Constantine Porphyrogenitus, the Byzantine emperor. Olga may have encountered Christians before, but she had never seen a Christian city, and Constantinople in the tenth century was the most glorious, most opulent city in all Christendom. Here, under circumstances that have not come down to us, Olga accepted the Christian faith and asked to be baptized. When she returned to Kiev, Olga built a church in her city and another at Pskov, all the while urging her people to become Christians. Very few were persuaded to convert from paganism, however. Perhaps they found it hard to believe that this brutal, bloody-minded woman was sincere when she extolled the virtues of turning the other cheek. Even members of her family rejected the faith. Her son and heir, Svyatoslav, dismissed Christianity with its loving, gentle

Jesus, as a religion for weaklings, completely unsuitable for a warrior people like the Rus.

Olga died disappointed by her failure to convert her country. In the years that followed her death and Svyatoslav's succession, the people of Rus showed no sign of abandoning their traditional pagan religion in favor of Christianity. When Svyatoslav died, he left his crown to his legitimate heir, Yaropolk. However, Svyatoslav's illegitimate son, Vladimir, believed he would make a better prince, so he assassinated his half-brother and seized the crown.

At Kiev Vladimir built an immense temple in which he set up statues of all the gods of Rus, as well as the gods of the neighboring tribes. He decided to consecrate the temple in the ancient manner— with human sacrifice. The victims he chose were Theodore and John, a father and son who were among the tiny handful of Christians living in Vladimir's realm.

Vladimir's lifestyle ran counter to Christianity in other ways as well: for example, he had seven wives and kept a harem of hundreds of women. As if all those women weren't enough, after assisting the Byzantine emperor Basil in a war against the Bulgars, Vladimir demanded as his reward the emperor's sister, Anna. The Byzantine aristocracy was outraged by the idea that an imperial princess should marry a barbarian; Anna herself was horrified by the thought of becoming Vladimir's eighth wife. Basil, however, felt that he had no choice other than to hand over his sister. Hoping to make the best of a bad situation, he insisted that Vladimir be baptized and give up his evil ways. Vladimir agreed, and the wedding took place immediately after his baptism.

No one expected Vladimir to keep his word, but when he returned to Kiev he gave clear signs that he had truly become a Christian. He dismantled the pagan temple; he dismissed his harem and his first seven wives; he sent bishops and priests to the cities and towns of Rus to preach the gospel; he gave generously to the poor, arranging for free meals to be served to the hungry and homeless every day. When Vladimir abolished the death penalty in his kingdom, even the Christian clergy were stunned; in the eleventh century no one considered capital punishment immoral.

Apparently when Vladimir was baptized the grace of God touched him and he truly repented. By the time of his death in 1015, Christianity was firmly established in Ukraine and was spreading into what is now Russia. Today both Olga and Vladimir are venerated as saints, and for introducing Christianity into Ukraine and Russia they have been given the title "Equal to the Apostles."

No Professor of Prayer

Father Cyril called on us early the next morning. He had not been able to persuade any other monks at the Pecherskaya Lavra to agree to an interview, but the abbot of St. Jonas Monastery nearby was willing to speak with us on-camera.

It was a short trip: within fifteen minutes we were at the monastery church in the heart of Kiev. Waiting for us was a young brother with very red hair, Father Jonas. He was the abbot, although I would guess he was only in his twenties. Our interview began with a conversation about monastic life during the Communist era, when monks who remained faithful to their vocation risked imprisonment in a gulag in Siberia or even death. Father Jonas observed that now that the Soviet Union has collapsed and religious persecution is becoming a distant memory, the monasteries are flourishing, with large numbers of men entering the religious life. The issue now, Father Jonas said, is "quantity, not quality." I asked him to explain.

"Maybe there were fewer monks [during the Communist era]," Father Jonas said, "but they were real monks; they were martyrs. They suffered a lot. And now there are more monks, but their quality is not the same." If Father Jonas was suggesting that today's monks lacked the fervor and commitment of their predecessors, I did not see it.

St. Jonas Monastery is small, with only twenty monks, all of them young. This may be intentional, since the monks of St. Jonas operate an outreach mission to the young people of Kiev.

"This monastery is located in the center of Kiev," Father Jonas said. "It's not like the monasteries which are in the suburbs or in some

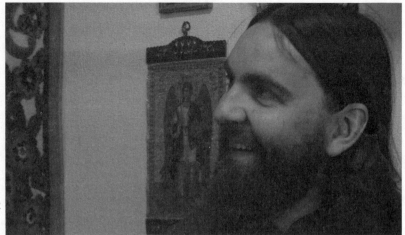

Photo by John Foster

Archdeacon Paisij of St. Jonas Monastery glows after
reciting the Jesus Prayer with us and for us.

villages, where the monks are more quiet, where they have more solitude. But in this monastery we try to reach the people of the city, to
bring them a message of peace. We support the activities of young
people; we visit hospitals; we visit the elderly in their homes often."

As he spoke, Father Jonas got out his mobile phone and made a
call. Soon thereafter another monk came around and led us inside
a dormitory, where he introduced us to Archdeacon Paisij. Another
young monk with very long hair and beard, Father Paisij welcomed
us but insisted that he was the wrong man to interview. "I am not a
professor of prayer!" he said. "I have nothing to say, except to repeat
what the Holy Fathers of the Church have said."

"But you practice prayer, and that's what a monk does, doesn't he?"
I asked him.

"I am not proud of myself," Father Paisij said. "I pray only in humility. One cannot be proud of praying."

As we spoke, Father Paisij led us to his cell. It was very tidy, with
everything neatly arranged, and many books on his shelves. "I try to
read a lot," he explained, "and the books, the works of the Holy Fathers, they help me to understand how to live, how to pray."

I asked him if he speaks directly with God, which I suspect he does; but humble man that he is, he denied it. God does communicate with us, Father Paisij said, but only through the Gospels and the teachings of the saints.

I tried a different tack. "What, then, is the way to happiness, Father?" I asked.

"In this life those people are happy who have Jesus Christ as a source of well-being and happiness," he replied. "You may have a lot of money, you may occupy a high position, but that will not make you happy in this life. You may have just a small cell, but if you communicate, if you talk to God, then you will be happy. Because happiness is being with God." He paused for a moment. "Because God is love." He paused again. "And where love is, there is no place for evil."

We were all silent for several minutes. Then Father Paisij reached over to a post next to his library shelf and took down a small circular leather rope. It was a loop about four inches long, with a leather cross dangling from it and about a hundred wooden dowels woven into the leather, like the rungs on a ladder. I recognized it as a *lestovka,* or "ladder," the traditional prayer rope of the Ukrainian and Russian Orthodox. The number of dowels varies from prayer rope to prayer rope, and the numbers have a mystical meaning: twelve dowels represent the apostles; thirty-nine represent the length in weeks of the pregnancy of Mary, the Mother of God; thirty-three represent the years of Christ's life on earth; and seventeen is the number of the prophets. Father Paisij handed the *lestovka* to me and said, in heavily accented English, "For you, friend." Tears welled up in my eyes. I was deeply moved and honored by Father Paisij's generosity.

Father John told me later that these prayer ropes are very old and quite rare; few monks have them anymore. I'm at a loss for words to describe how much this gift means to me. I carry it with me everywhere now. I often try to practice the Jesus Prayer with it—not so much to keep count, but to keep my mind focused.

It was hard to say goodbye to Father Paisij, but before we left, we prayed with him for a few moments. "I kiss the cross," Father Paisij said. "I pray to God to save the whole world."

One Thousand Years of Saints

Outside Father Paisij's cell another young monk, who introduced himself as Father Maxim, was waiting for us. He led us through a long park with a botanical garden. Suddenly, it began to rain. Seeing our concern for our equipment, Father Maxim led us quickly to a brick church that was under construction on the site of what he told us had been the Zverinetsky Skete, a sister monastic community to St. Jonas. "This is the skete," he explained. "This is a new church. It is being built because the old [one] was destroyed by the Soviets." The rain intensified and we needed better shelter than a partially built church. Father Maxim ran down a flight of steps, beckoning for us to follow, and took us through a metal door set in the side of a very large mound. We followed the young monk down more steps until we reached a tunnel. There Father Maxim lit a candle, illuminating an old, dark icon of Christ, which he kissed. Turning to us he said, "Welcome to the Zverinetsky caves!" He said it with glee. This was his surprise for us.

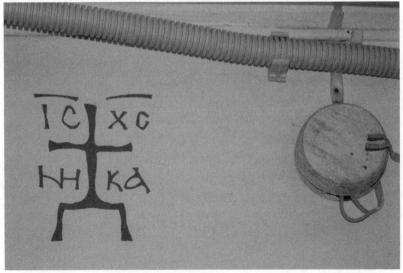

The ancient symbol of the Zverinetsky Skete, sister monastic community of the St. Jonas Monastery, Kiev. It depicts both Jesus Christ and the Cross in one. This symbol is all over Kiev; we even spotted it on a car bumper!

The Zverinetsky caves are older than the caves of the Pecherskaya Lavra, but they are less well known. They are also in their original condition—dirt floors, dirt tunnels, and no electricity. Before we began our exploration of the caves, Father Maxim spontaneously chanted an ancient hymn in Ukrainian. It was an unforgettable moment.

He then showed us the cells of the monks. There were piles of bones in most of them, though not neatly wrapped in shrouds or encased in protective glass as we had seen at the Pecherskaya Lavra. Here the relics of a thousand years of saints lay untouched, undisturbed, in the place where those men had lived and died. The skull of one saint was giving off myrrh, but there were no lines of pilgrims to venerate it—only us.

These tunnels were not easy to negotiate. Often I had to crouch down because of a low ceiling, or squeeze myself through a narrow passage. Father Maxim led us to a primitive underground chapel, furnished only with two stones for chairs and a stone table for an altar. I had the feeling that very few people have ever had the privilege to be in that ancient holy place.

We spent several hours in the Zverinetsky caves, but they went by quickly. When we returned to the staircase, but before we left the tunnel, Father Maxim offered a prayer of thanksgiving to the holy fathers of the Zverinetsky caves. Then we climbed the stairs and stepped out into sunshine, the rain having moved on.

As we walked with Father Maxim, he told us how pleased the brothers were that we were making a film about prayer, that we were bringing the message of Jesus Christ to the world. Before we parted, he gave us gifts of incense, a CD of the monks of St. Jonas singing Christmas hymns in the caves, and a wonderful poster of the seven deadly sins, portrayed by monks in cassocks.

The Princess's Monastery

After our remarkable experience in the Zverinetsky caves we climbed back into the van and headed to the Pokrovsky Monastery, a convent several miles outside the city. When we arrived, we found that we

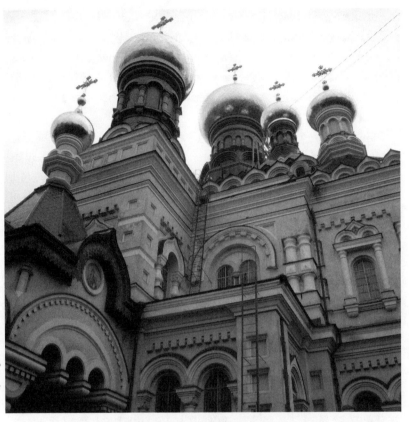

Photo by Dwight Grimm

The Cathedral of St. Nicholas at the Pokrovsky Monastery in Kiev, Ukraine, founded in 1889 by Princess Alexandra Petrovna.

were the only visitors. We encountered a few nuns washing floors and cleaning the Church of the Holy Virgin, but they went about their duties, paying no mind to us. Even when we began to film, the sisters did not react. We had always had tremendous difficulty convincing any nuns to appear in our movie, but not here.

Pokrovsky Monastery was founded in 1889 by Princess Alexandra Petrovna, the sister-in-law of Tsar Alexander II. She became a nun here herself—in fact, she became abbess—and used her fortune to fund the day-to-day operation of the monastery. The main church, the Cathedral of St. Nicholas, is delightful—sea-green walls, sky-blue roof, glowing gold onion domes. The day it was consecrated in 1896, the princess's nephew Nicholas and his wife Alexandra—the last tsar and tsarina of Russia—attended the ceremony. Pokrovsky Monastery fell on hard times in 1925, when the Communist government expelled the nuns and took over the convent buildings for secular purposes. One building became a police station; another became a radio repair shop.

As we wandered around, a sister came to welcome us to the convent. She introduced herself as Sister Angelina and explained that she had been sent by the mother superior. I asked her if she herself would agree to be interviewed; Sister Angelina said she would be delighted. And so we sat down and began to talk, as always, about prayer.

"We pray during services," Sister Angelina said; "we pray when we fulfill our tasks, being obedient, and we pray for ourselves, and we pray for our relatives, and we pray for the whole world. Everything we do, we do it with prayer. Before doing something we say, 'God help me' or 'God bless me,' and when we're finished doing something we say, 'Thank you, God.'"

I asked her if she and her fellow nuns prayed the Jesus Prayer. "We pray this Jesus Prayer; we try to do it all the time. But we have not reached the level really, that level to pray it constantly. Now I would be happy to have this gift of constantly praying the Jesus Prayer, because it is a gift from God. It comes from God."

I asked Sister Angelina another question. "How does God speak, Sister? How does God feel in your heart?"

"God is love," she replied. "God is quietness, God is peace; and if I feel love and peace in my heart, I know that I am close to God."

Sister Angelina is the supervisor of the convent's bakery, and she invited us to see where she works. Every day they make *prosphora* (Greek for "that which is offered"), or Holy Eucharist bread, as well as thousands of little hand-stamped pieces of bread called *antidora* that are distributed to anyone who visits the church. These little breads are blessed, but they are not the Eucharist that the Orthodox receive in Holy Communion. Sister Angelina introduced us to her co-workers, the sisters who mixed the hundreds of pounds of dough, shaped and kneaded it, placed it on special racks, and baked it. After

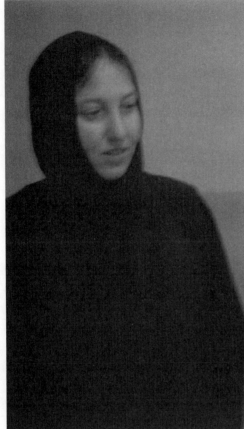

Photo by Dwight Grimm

Sister Angelina of Pokrovsky Monastery, Kiev. She is the head of the convent's bakery, making *prosphora* (Greek for "that which is offered"), or Holy Eucharist bread, as well as *antidora,* individual little breads that are distributed to anyone who visits the church.

we finished filming, she gave us bags full of warm, delicious *antidora* to take with us.

But Sister Angelina's generosity was not over yet. She took us into a little dining room and served us three kinds of homemade soup. One of them was borscht, the second a delicious potato broth, and the third a cabbage and vegetable soup cooked with a ham hock. We were greatly appreciative; we had been on the move all that day and had had no time to eat.

As she walked us back to our minivan, Sister Angelina told us that the convent had once had a thriving hospital, founded by Princess Alexandra herself when she established the convent. It was destroyed

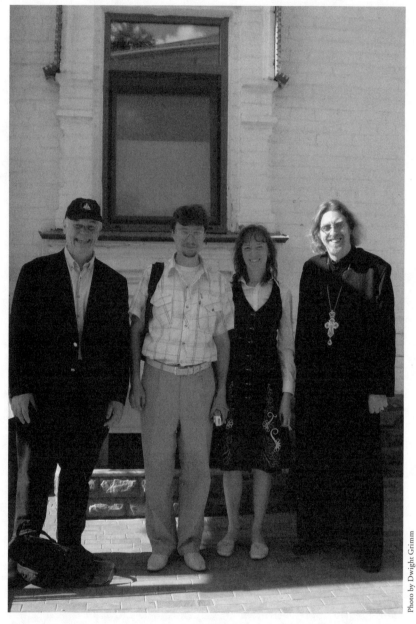

Father John and I say goodbye to Kiev and the Pecherskaya Lavra, and to our wonderful guides and translators Anthony and Helen Vovchenko. They were just married when we were there and have since had a baby boy. They named him Cyril, after the great priest and monk Cyril Hovorun, who introduced them—whom we also interviewed (and who served as our host at the Pecherskaya Lavra).

during the Communist era, and the nuns do not have the funds to rebuild the hospital. They hope to do so someday, however. I pray that they will, as they are exceptionally kind and loving people.

. . .

We had known bountiful kindness and generosity during our days in Kiev, and our visit concluded with a supreme example of it. Our guide, Igor Issayev, director of the American Business Center in Ukraine, invited us to dinner at a wonderful restaurant called Khutorets, on a floating barge on the Dnieper River. We were joined by the manager of the chain of restaurants (the Royal Card) that owns Khutorets. This is the finest restaurant in all of Ukraine, and we were special guests. Igor led us to a private dining room, where we were served course after course of delicious Ukrainian delicacies. At times like this, I am glad to not be a monk. Nonetheless, before eating, we all prayed and thanked God for all his blessings—most particularly, for our astonishing week in Kiev.

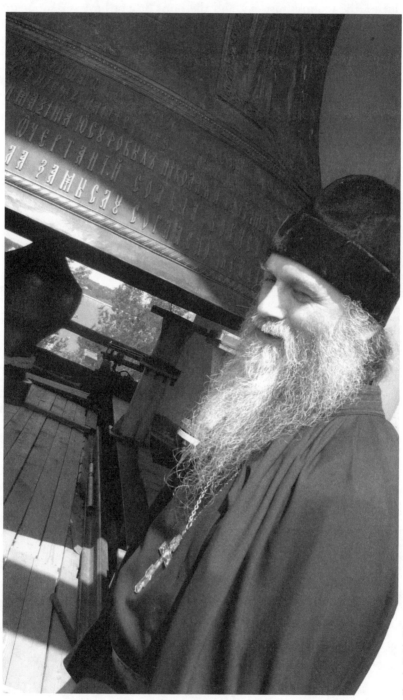

8

The Jesus Prayer amid
the Grandeur of Russia

RUSSIA CAN BE SUMMED UP in one word—grand. Everything is big: it is an enormous country that covers nearly 6.6 million square miles, with a population of approximately 142 million; it is a country of large cities, massive buildings, huge plazas, expansive churches and cathedrals, a vast and powerful government, and 100 million members of the Russian Orthodox Church.

Under the Soviet government the Russian Orthodox Church suffered dreadfully. Countless numbers of bishops, monks, nuns, seminarians, and the ordinary faithful were deported to labor camps or killed outright. Many churches, monasteries, and convents were expropriated for secular purposes (and their treasures looted), while others were abandoned and still others wantonly destroyed.

In Moscow the Soviets used the Danilovsky Monastery as a holding pen for dissidents who were about to be executed. The seminary

Opposite: Father Jacob with the world's largest bell, in the bell tower at Sergiyev Posad Monastery in Russia. It is about to ring an ear-shattering and soul-shaking announcement of Patriarch Kirill's arrival. It takes twelve large bell-ringers to make it sound.

next door was converted into an orphanage for the dissidents' children. The Soviets had planned to destroy the monastery's bells, but an American businessman stepped in and bought them, donating them to Harvard University. A year before we visited Russia, Harvard returned the bells to the reopened Danilovsky Monastery. They ring again every hour, and in the context of the monastery's history, the sound is particularly sweet.

Waiting to welcome us in Moscow was Zinoviy Chesnokov, our twenty-something Russian Orthodox Church escort and translator. Zinoviy is a student at the Moscow Theological Academy, where he is studying to be a priest. He lives about forty-five miles northeast of the city at Russia's most important monastery, Sergiyev Posad, the one-and-only sacred site where we would be filming in Russia. Zinoviy is a serious young man, with a modest and humble demeanor; he is also capable, personable, smart, and well organized. He had a minivan waiting at the airport to take us to the Danilovsky Monastery, where we would spend two nights; the next day we would take a day trip to

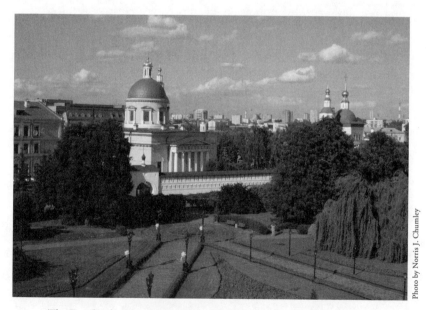

Photo by Norris J. Chumley

The Danilovsky Monastery in the center of Moscow, Russia—home of
His Eminence Kirill, patriarch of Moscow and all Russia.

our destination: Sergiyev Posad. Zinoviy was the advance man for the Moscow Patriarchate, which cleared away every obstacle and proved to be of enormous help in gaining access to this famous monastery.

Before traveling to any monasteries or meeting any monks or nuns, we wanted to capture images of some very old and famous artwork: an icon of Christ, an icon of the Holy Trinity, and a painting of St. Sergius of Radonezh (c. 1320–1392), the monk who founded Sergiyev Posad. All of them are displayed in the state-owned Tretyakov Gallery in Moscow. These extraordinary examples of Russian sacred art were something both Father John and I very much wanted to see, so we made a beeline from the airport to the museum.

Even the Tretyakov had a government-style bureaucracy. In spite of all our advance preparations, there were piles of paperwork to complete, countless officials who had to approve our request, layer upon layer of security guards to clear us. It took us four hours to make our way through clearance, and by that time the museum was ready to close. Finally, escorted by a posse of guards, clutching a stack of permissions, Father John, Zinoviy, and I rendezvoused with our cinematographers, Dwight Grimm and Jack Foster, at the icons.

As we stood in front of the *Mandylion,* the face of Christ painted by the genius iconographer Andrei Rublev in the late fourteenth or early fifteenth century, all the vicissitudes of securing permissions and visas, all the hardships of travel and transport melted away. I had seen this icon of the face of Christ in many books, and I even have a reproduction of it painted by Father John's talented wife, the iconographer Eileen McGuckin. Being in the presence of the original was an indescribable experience. It was like being with Jesus Christ in person. There was at once a feeling of otherworldliness and immediate presence. Christ was among us, as the monks often say. When I looked into the eyes of the icon, I felt him looking directly back at me, even though the eyes appeared to look to my left. I knew that this indirect gaze was particularly Byzantine, as it was considered inappropriate or even blasphemous for the subject of an icon to make eye contact.

This is a famous and revered icon for good reason. In the sacred image, the *Mandylion* icon of Jesus Christ, the presence of God in His

Uncreated Energies may be strongly felt. Was it the initial blessings of the priests that charged it up? Perhaps its great power comes from the veneration of millions of believers for whom this icon has been an object of great love and reverence for many centuries. Certainly it is an outstanding example of artistry and history. To me it is all of the above, but at that moment, standing next to it in faraway Moscow, I felt the supreme love of God with us.

The icon's title comes from the Byzantine Greek word *mandylion,* which means "cloth." An ancient legend tells of an artist who went to Jesus and asked his permission to paint his portrait. Jesus agreed, but the artist found that in spite of all his skill and repeated attempts, he could not capture on canvas the face of Christ. Jesus took a cloth, pressed it to his face, and then handed the fabric to the artist. Imprinted on the cloth was a perfect portrait of Christ, which is known as the *Mandylion.* Because of the miraculous manner by which the original was made, the *Mandylion* is often referred to as "not painted by human hands." There are many reproductions of the original *Mandylion,* but none is as great as the *Mandylion* of Andrei Rublev.

Rublev's icon, which measures about three feet by three feet, was intended for religious processions. On holy days or "feasts," it was mounted on a pole and carried through the streets with crowds of priests and parishioners following behind. The procession symbolized that Christ is the Head of the Church, and the faithful walk humbly in his footsteps.

Next, we were led through a maze of interlinking stairways and doorways to a church adjacent to the Tretyakov Gallery—a church where perhaps the most famous of all the Rublev icons resides, the *Troitsa* (or *Holy Trinity*). This is a large icon depicting the three angels who appeared to St. Abraham and St. Sarah as recorded in Genesis 18. Traditionally, the three angels have been interpreted as the Father, the Son, and the Holy Spirit—the Three Persons of the Holy Trinity. Other icons that depict this scriptural event often include the figure of Abraham, Sarah peeking out of the family tent, and other objects, but Rublev has reduced the scene to what is essential—the angels— with only a tree (one of the oaks of Mamre, mentioned in Genesis

18:1), to anchor the scene to the biblical text. As I gazed at the icon, I once again felt a palpable flow of energy that is impossible to describe.

Father John told me that the late patriarch of the Russian Orthodox Church, His Eminence Patriarch Alexy II, as he lay on his deathbed in 2008, sent a request to the Russian government asking for the return of the *Troitsa* icon to the Orthodox Church. A few days after he fell asleep in the Lord, government authorities decided that this was not possible, citing concerns for the care and maintenance of a priceless national treasure. But the government granted the Orthodox Church a concession: once a year, on the Feast of the Holy Trinity, the Tretyakov would move the icon into the adjacent church for three days. By luck or grace we happened to be in Russia on that occasion and were able to film it in its rightful place.

Finally, before we had to leave the Tretyakov, we were able to photograph another fantastic work of art, the *Vision of the Youth Bartholomew,* by Mikhail Vasilyevich Nesterov (painted 1889–1890). The painting depicts an event from the life of St. Sergius of Radonezh. When he was a little boy named Bartholomew, he asked an elderly monk to teach him the alphabet. The old monk, cloaked in a black cassock and holding icons and some ABC cards, dominates the painted scene. In the background is a church with large onion domes, perhaps a reference to the monastery St. Sergei (as he is known to most Russians) would found, the Sergiyev Posad. Studying this painting, I felt even more excited to visit Sergiyev Posad and learn more of St. Sergei.

Sergei's Village

We all enjoyed a good night's sleep in Moscow at the patriarch's hotel, the Danilovsky, which hosts visiting bishops and clergy. The next morning, as planned, our minivan carried us and our gear to St. Sergei's monastery.

It would be difficult to overstate St. Sergei's importance in the religious, cultural, and national life of Russia. He is the most significant of the *pustiniky,* the men of the wilderness, monks as energetic as they were holy, who revived Russian culture and Russian monastic life after the devastating Mongol invasion of the thirteenth century. In 1335, when he was about twenty years old, Bartholomew and his older brother Istvan went into the woods to a place called Makovka, where they built a hut and a chapel and lived as hermits. Bartholomew, in keeping with an old tradition of those who have entered the religious life, took a new name—Sergius. The brothers had not been at Makovka long when Istvan decided that he was not suited to the rigors of a hermitage and left for a monastery in Moscow. Sergius remained, and soon other devout men joined, building their huts around the little rustic chapel dedicated to the Holy Trinity. From this small community grew the great monastery of St. Sergei and the Holy Trinity, known in Russia as Sergiyev Posad, meaning "Sergei's village."

Russians revere St. Sergei as a peacemaker and a patriot: he resolved disputes between squabbling Russian princes, and Prince Dmitry Donskoy attributed his victory over the Tatars in 1380 to the prayers of St. Sergei. And St. Sergei enjoys another distinction: he is the first Russian saint to have received an apparition of the Blessed Virgin Mary.

It was about a two-and-a-half-hour ride north/northeast through Moscow and its suburbs, then into birch forests, to get to the monastery and the charming little town adjacent to it. You can see the bell tower of the monastery from many miles away. Then, as we came closer, the amazingly beautiful blue and gold onion domes of the Assumption Cathedral and the golden domes of the Holy Trinity Cathedral and Refectory Church came into view.

There is no agreement among historians as to why Russian churches are crowned with distinctive onion-shaped domes. Some say the reason is practical: snow cannot collect on them. Others claim it is a kind of tribute to onions, Russia's largest crop. Still others say the domes were inspired by the bulbous domes of Islamic mosques and minarets. A more poetic view holds that the onion domes are meant to resemble burning candles. A dome's color is significant, too: the golden ones are mirrors of the universe, reflecting light from God;

blue domes with gold stars mirror the stars in God's firmament; green, blue, and gold together represent the Holy Trinity. The number of the domes above a church has meaning as well: a single dome signifies Jesus Christ; four represent Christ and his three closest apostles—Peter, James, and John; three domes represent the Holy Trinity. Atop each dome rises the three-barred Russian cross. The topmost bar of the cross represents the *titulus,* or title-board, which Pontus Pilate ordered hung above the head of Jesus. Pilate's inscription read, "Jesus of Nazareth, King of the Jews." In the Russian Orthodox Church,

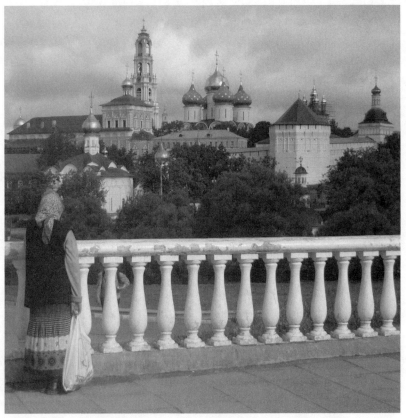

Photo by Dwight Grimm

A parishioner stops at a scenic overlook to view the great Sergiyev Posad Monastery and the magnificent onion domes of Holy Spirit Church (*left foreground*), the bell tower (*tallest*), and Assumption Cathedral (*center*).

that mocking inscription is replaced with a Christian declaration of faith: "The King of Glory." The second bar of a Russian cross is the crosspiece to which Christ's hands were nailed. The third, diagonal bar represents the brace to which Christ's feet were nailed.

We pulled over at a scenic overlook and set up our cameras for the first panoramic shots of the monastery—the gigantic walled fortress, the watchtowers rising above the battlements, and the countless churches and chapels and monastic buildings within that are home to approximately 300 monks.

Sergiyev Posad is by far the largest and most important monastery in all of Russia, and one of the biggest in the world. It was the home of the Russian patriarch until 1988, when he moved to the more centrally located Danilovsky Monastery in the center of Moscow. It is very different from any of the other monasteries we visited—it is like a small city enclosed in a high circular fortress. There are several gates, but only one main entry point. From the cobblestone plaza in front it's only a short walk to the entry, past a gigantic statue of St. Sergei. There's also (curiously) a statue of Lenin. I'd have thought that would have been torn down long ago, given the history of the monastery. The Lenin-led Bolsheviks closed the monastery in 1917, sent the monks to labor camps, and confiscated the relics of St. Sergei, which they displayed in what we might call an anti-religion museum. In 1945, as part of the Soviet Union's victory celebrations at the end of World War II, Joseph Stalin returned the monastery to the Russian Orthodox Church. The following year regular liturgical services were restored at the Assumption Cathedral.

In addition to being a thriving monastic community and a goal for pilgrims who come to venerate the relics of St. Sergei, Sergiyev Posad houses four major church schools: the Moscow Theological Academy, a seminary, a school of iconography, and a school of church music. In addition to its many churches and chapels, the monastery has an awesome museum filled with inestimable treasures, including sacred vessels, sacred vestments, and rare icons.

The Holy Trinity Cathedral, built in 1422, is where the relics of St. Sergei are enshrined in front of an iconostasis. Many of the icons in the screen are the work of Andrei Rublev. Prayer is unceasing in this holy place, with an unending stream of pilgrims lining up to venerate the saint's shrine and ask for his intercession.

During our time at Sergiyev Posad we saw thousands upon thousands of pilgrims seemingly from all over the world. Perhaps it is because we were there during the Feast of the Holy Trinity, also known as Pentecost, the most important holy day on the Russian Orthodox calendar, after Easter and Christmas. Zinoviy, as a student and resident, acted as our guide and took us into places where ordinary pilgrims could not go. He also seemed to know all the professors, priests, and monks, often stopping to exchange a kiss of peace with them. It was Zinoviy who arranged for us to interview one of the monks' spiritual leaders, Father Jacob.

Interview in a Bell Tower

We met Father Jacob near the outrageously long line of pilgrims waiting to get inside the cathedral to pay homage to St. Sergei. The location had lots of human interest, but it was too noisy. We asked Father Jacob if there was a quiet place where we could record. He smiled widely and pointed skyward. "Heaven?" I thought to myself, until I looked up. He meant the enormous bell tower. I laughed and said, "Yeah!" Father Jacob patted me on the back and motioned for Father John, Zinoviy, and our crew—Jack and Dwight—to follow him.

He took us into the gift shop, where he unlocked and led us through an unmarked door and into the base of the tower. Then up and up we climbed, following a circular stairway in pitch darkness, lugging our equipment with us. The fathers in their cassocks climbed slowly ahead of us, careful not to lose their footing. It was a relief to see daylight and come out at last at the top of the bell tower. Father Jacob grinned from ear to ear. "Here is all of Russia before our eyes!" he exclaimed. We were indeed at a very high point, higher than the glowing gold onion domes of the churches. I thought to myself that if I reached out, I would touch clouds.

Father Jacob had a particular interest in our film because, as he explained, he, too, was a film producer. He had been the chaplain of the Sergiyev Posad monastery at the South Pole and had made several films there. The monks keep the scientists company during their long winter expeditions. And as the South Pole is a silent place, it is excellent for monastic life. Three years ago he returned to Sergiyev Posad.

Father Jacob spoke to us about monasticism being the core of the Christian life, but noted that all Christians who devote their lives to the vocation assigned to them by God are living a kind of monastic life. For monks and nuns, as for people in the world, he explained, "the love is the same, the commandments are the same, and practically . . . the way is the same, the way to the heavenly Father through the love of Jesus Christ, his beloved Son, who became sacrificed for our salvation."

Father Jacob said that he believed the life of the monks was much easier than the life of Christians out in the world. People encounter so many daily obstacles and challenges in the world, he said, but the monks have only to pray. "My heart, my feelings, my soul, my body, my brains—they belong to Christ," Father Jacob said. "That's why I'm not afraid of the circumstances of this world—of temptations, of sorrows, of difficulties." Temptations and troubles are nothing, he assured us, when we are united with Jesus Christ through the Jesus Prayer. "That is why we are free with God. You see, it's a very optimistic feeling." He again smiled from ear to ear. The light of Christ was in his smile.

When Father John asked him specifically about the Jesus Prayer, Father Jacob taught us that it is a "foundation . . . the main bedrock of life." Father John commented that he felt "as if there is no prayer within [many Christian communities]." Father Jacob replied that it is a "tragedy of many Christians[;] . . . there is a loss of the treasury of pure Christianity." The Jesus Prayer to him, and to the Russian Church, he believes, is life itself: "It is the new day, and the new appreciation of every moment of our being before the face of God."

Prayer, Father Jacob explained, is central to being a Christian; it offers both a method of direct communication with God and an unfolding of spiritual life. The Jesus Prayer is something that he and his fellow monks practice every moment of every day, but he felt that it is not exclusive to monasticism. He encouraged us to pray regularly, too, along with the monks.

At that point, the bells began to ring, one after another, rising to a crescendo of ringing in every conceivable tone. Father Jacob yelled out, "This is the exclamation point to our talk about the Jesus Prayer! Come with me, now!"

He grabbed my hand, and I grabbed a little camera from Dwight and ran downstairs, back down the pitch-dark circular stairway. A flight or two down he opened a little door and we stepped onto a wooden platform. There I saw a dozen large men, all gathered beneath and beside an enormous bronze bell that must have measured at least ten feet wide and eight feet high. Inside hung the bronze clapper, about the size of a six-foot-tall man. Shouting over the clanging of the bells, Father Jacob yelled to me, "This is the world's largest bell. It weighs seventy-two [metric] tons." I watched as the men, six on each side, pulled a massive rope back and forth; they had gotten the clapper in motion, but it had not yet struck the sides of the giant bell.

"Patriarch Kirill is about to arrive," Father Jacob shouted. I followed his gaze over the side of the railing; below us thousands of bishops, monks, and pilgrims were lined up, waiting for the arrival of His Eminence, the Patriarch of All Russia, who was coming to celebrate the Divine Liturgy the next day.

Suddenly, I heard walkie-talkies emitting voices speaking in urgent Russian. The dozen bell-ringers gave extra-heavy heaves on the ropes and the clapper finally made contact with the bell. It wasn't like ringing at all; it was an intensely low-pitched vibration that increased exponentially with each *dong*. After three or four strikes, the vibration began to be almost unbearably intense. Because I was only a few feet from the bell, the sound wasn't so much entering through my ears as it was penetrating through my bones and sinew, straight to the edges

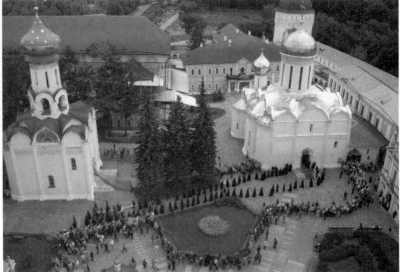

Photo by John A. McGuckin

We watch from our perch high atop the bell tower at Sergiyev Posad Monastery as His Eminence Kirill, patriarch of Moscow and all Russia, arrives the afternoon before the Feast of the Holy Trinity. Many monks, bishops, and parishioners delight in his presence. The bells ring out to announce his arrival.

of my soul. Growing louder and louder, deeper and deeper, it touched me to the core, and I began to weep uncontrollably. The dozen bell-ringers hauled on the ropes with all their strength for another five minutes; then they simply let go. It took a good half an hour for the bell to stop vibrating. I was completely speechless through the whole experience.

Father Jacob came over to me, shaking his head from side to side in full understanding of what had just happened to me, saying, "You will never forget this moment as long as you live." Later, another monk said to me, "Bells are the voice of God."

A Continual Festival

That afternoon Zinoviy took us on a tour of the Moscow Theological Academy, including its beautiful museum full of icons, sacred vestments, mementos of many patriarchs, ancient church jewels, and holy

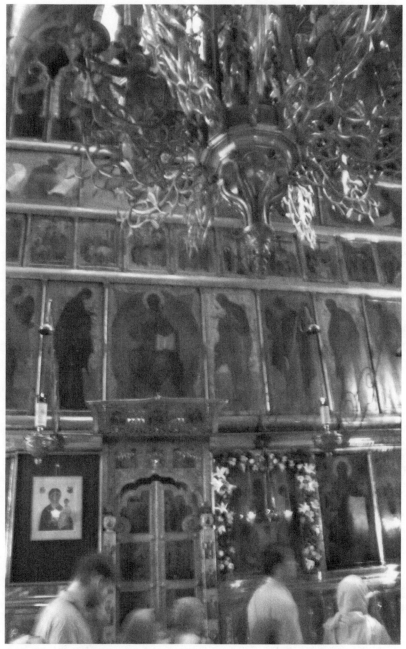

Photo by Norris J. Chumley

The magnificent iconostasis of the Holy Trinity Cathedral, Sergiyev Posad Monastery. Note the Rublev icons on the second level above the door, masterpieces still in use in the church by a steady stream of parishioners flowing by.

relics. He took us to the old refectory, a magnificent and very old building once used to feed large crowds.

Finally, like every other pilgrim at the monastery, we made our way to the Cathedral of the Holy Trinity to visit St. Sergei and personally thank him for our visit. It's a continual festival in that church, as if St. Sergei were still alive and well, eager to greet the throngs of pilgrims lined up beneath the sublime icons of the iconostasis.

Zinoviy used his status as a student and our official assistant to take us into chapels that are off-limits to most pilgrims. We saw relics of all kinds, belonging to saints and clergy from many centuries, as well as thousands of icons and paintings. Zinoviy showed us the side door to the main church, still marred by bullet holes sustained during the Bolshevik takeover. I could sense the oppression and terror of that era, mixed with the joy of the monks and students over the glorious renewal of their monastery.

After a full day rich in unforgettable experiences, it was time to return to our quarters in Moscow for the night.

Divine Liturgy with the Patriarch

The next morning, very early, we were back again in our minivan. After traveling by a different route through a beautiful birch forest, we arrived back at Sergiyev Posad along with thousands of other pilgrims. Thanks to Zinoviy, we escaped the crowds and were escorted through a different entryway into the Assumption Cathedral—one that brought us to the front of the church where the Divine Liturgy was about to begin.

There was a section reserved for large cameras, probably twenty of them already in place, with their operators all lined up. John "Jack" Foster, one of our cinematographers, took a place right at the front, next to a candle-stand maintained by a little girl, perhaps only ten years old, wearing a pretty headscarf. Father John, Dwight, and I were on the other side of the sanctuary with our additional camera. Fortunately, I'm tall, so I could hold it up and get high-perspective shots over the heads of the worshippers. The church was completely full, with thousands of adults and children crowded in, all standing shoulder to shoulder and craning their necks to get a glimpse of the liturgy. I've never seen so many people in a church at one time.

Assumption Cathedral was built in the late sixteenth century by the Russian tsar Ivan the Terrible in thanksgiving for his victory at Kazan over the last of the powerful Mongol Tatars that once controlled Russia. It is a magnificent church, crowned with five domes. Painted inside the main dome is a majestic icon of Christ looking down on the congregation. The walls and columns of the church are covered with icons and murals of saints and martyrs, painted in intensely rich colors and embossed with gold leaf. The iconostasis is another treasure, filled with rare icons and covered with more gold. Suspended over our heads were giant chandeliers, each illuminated with hundreds of bulbs. Candle-stands were everywhere, with beeswax candles all aflame, each symbolizing the light of God's love, and a hope and prayer for those afar, or in distress, or asleep in the Lord.

The center of the altar area was filled with big pots of living birch trees in delicate green leaf, in honor of the saint of the Russian birch forest, St. Sergei. There were thousands of fresh flowers as well: lilies and orchids of every conceivable size, color, and shape. Just in front of us was an instantly recognizable icon covered in white lilies on a special stand: Rublev's *Holy Trinity*! This was not the original icon, of course; we'd seen that in Moscow. As noted earlier, the agreement between the Russian government and the Russian Orthodox Church permits Rublev's icon to be displayed only in the church adjacent to the Tretyakov Gallery. The Sergiyev Posad is several hours away from Moscow—too great a distance to put at risk such a fragile treasure as Rublev's icon. What was presented to the faithful in the church of Sergiyev Posad was a most accurately painted reproduction, not a photograph. One by one members of the congregation stepped forward to venerate it, kissing the feet of the three angels.

From off in the distance we heard the sound of a single monk's prayers. The crowd of thousands hushed. This went on for several minutes; then a choir began—actually, two *bolshoi* (big) choirs on either side of the iconostasis, singing the most exquisite harmonies.

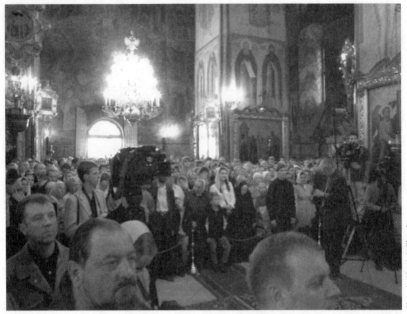

Thousands of believers and parishioners and dozens of
television cameras crowd Assumption Cathedral at Sergiyev
Posad Monastery for the Feast of the Holy Trinity.

Suddenly the golden doors of the iconostasis opened wide, revealing the light-filled Holy of Holies. Out came dozens of priests, deacons, and bishops who formed two parallel lines along the red carpet leading to the altar.

Then we heard the tinkling of bells, followed by the deep boom of the gigantic bronze bell, which radiated through the church. Shortly thereafter, a white-bearded man appeared wearing white-and-green-bejeweled vestments and a black-and-gold-rimmed miter that resembled a crown. It was Patriarch Kirill, flanked by a dozen security guards and followed by dozens of bishops. As he passed, the crowds bowed. Kirill's bearing, and the slow, careful steps he took as he approached the altar, convinced me that if he were an ordinary layman wearing ordinary street clothes, he would still be a remarkable person.

This was the most elaborate liturgy I'd ever experienced—certainly significantly different from the liturgies at St. Catherine's, Vatopedi, or Rohia, all of which had been much more modest. This Divine Liturgy was extremely formal, highly polished, and lavish, no doubt because of the unique combination of the feast day, the setting, and the presence of the patriarch. The clergy who attended Kirill performed their parts of the liturgy perfectly and with absolute precision. No one was ever out of place; no one made the least mistake in his chants. And when the clergy sang, their voices were heavenly.

The liturgy lasted several hours, and we were able to film sections of each part, from multiple angles. The service included an installation of a new priest, something I had never before witnessed. The priests, bishops, and patriarch actually grabbed the initiate monk by the arm and pulled him into the altar area. Father John whispered in my ear, "This is a typically Russian form of ordination, Norris. No one theoretically *wants* to become a public servant; the clergy determine that a priest is to be appointed and the candidate is pulled into the job by the arm!" I found this fascinating; and certainly it makes sense that the priesthood would be the kind of all-consuming and difficult job that your colleagues would have to "pull" you into. The ceremony dramatizes the belief that a man does not volunteer to be a priest; he is called to this vocation by God, and it is a call he cannot refuse. From the day of his ordination on, the priest's life is no longer entirely his own; henceforth he lives in service to others and in service to Christ's Church. But to see this so literally enacted in a church service, with robed and bejeweled clergy yanking a young candidate, was an experience.

At one point the liturgy stopped cold and Patriarch Kirill stepped out from the Holy Doors and began to preach to the crowd. I don't understand Russian, so I have no idea what he was saying, yet his voice was so commanding, his tone so compelling that I was mesmerized. His bearing was formal and serious; there were no smiles, no moments of levity, although occasionally he raised his voice considerably. It was a magisterial sermon, pure business.

After the service we hurried outside, where people of all kinds had gathered, waiting for a glimpse of the patriarch. After several minutes, bells began to ring again; the long line of security officials, bishops, and deacons came out the front door, followed by His Eminence. He processed through the crowd so that everyone assembled could see him.

Meanwhile, many people noticed Father John in his black cassock, wearing the gold cross that had been given to him by Metropolitan (now Patriarch of Romania) Daniel. As he wandered approachably through the crowds, they stopped him to ask for a blessing, kissing his hand and bowing. Obliging, Father John said a prayer in English over each of them and made the sign of the cross on their heads.

About an hour after the conclusion of the Divine Liturgy, when the area outside Assumption Cathedral was almost empty of pilgrims, I spied Father Jacob at the top of the bell tower sitting alone, looking out upon all of Russia, praying the Jesus Prayer by himself, in silence.

. . .

Months later, back in the United States, when all our footage had been assembled and the translated transcription of that Divine Liturgy had been delivered, I was quite moved and delighted to read what His Eminence Patriarch Kirill had said in his sermon:

God has no past, present, or future; he is beyond time and space. By the power of the Holy Spirit, through the sacramental mysteries, we too can overcome time and space, even the gravity of this physical world, for in a mystery we truly share in the Passion, the Cross, the Resurrection, the Ascension, [and the] exaltation and awesome Second Coming of Christ. The mystery of salvation takes place in the Church by the power of the Holy Spirit, and by that power everything that Christ has achieved becomes present to us in that community, becomes real for each human being in their life, regardless of the difference in time and place. By the power of the Holy Spirit, in the mystery of prayer, Christ's Church, and the mystery of the Eucharist, we come into contact with the divine life itself, the very life of heaven. Even though we are on earth, we touch the very kingdom of God.

Patriarch Kirill brings together the mysteries of the Jesus Prayer, and of all creation and human existence, when he explains in his sermon that it is through the Holy Spirit that we are first brought to the recognition of God's existence in us, in others, and in his creation. Through the mysteries of the sacraments (particularly the Holy Eucharist), we come into contact with God the Father, with Jesus Christ, and with the Holy Spirit and enter the kingdom of heaven. And we do so while we are still on earth!

We feel a "presence" of God at first; we receive a glimpse of the likeness of God that fills us with both joy and the desire to know God more fully. It is not enough, though, to only feel or see this image or likeness. It is important to take this awareness of God into your life and experience and express God in everything you do. Even though we are human beings in a physical world, we are also reflections of God through the Holy Spirit. It is this gift of the Holy Spirit inside us that is the vehicle for us to not only connect with God but to be guided by him in all our senses, ideas, emotions, works, and actions.

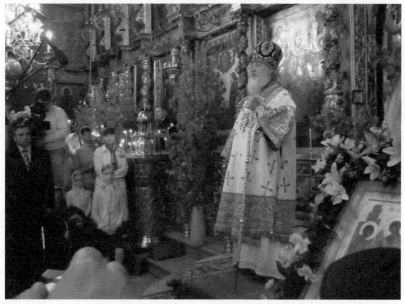

Photo by John A. McGuckin

His Eminence Kirill gives his sermon during the Feast of the Holy Trinity at Assumption Cathedral, Sergiyev Posad Monastery.

We are human and limited by physical constraints and boundaries, yet through the power of the Holy Spirit, we participate in eternity. Patriarch Kirill explained it beautifully for me in the words from the translated transcription of his sermon:

> *It is in the incarnated person of Jesus Christ, both God and divine human being, that we can go much, much deeper into the mystery of life, and of our purpose as human beings. God, our Creator and Father of All, takes human form in the person of his Son, Jesus Christ. This infusion of the Holy Spirit, which comes for the purpose of bringing us to God, becomes completely tangible in Christ, as God in human form. In the Church, God is present in the Holy Spirit, and in Jesus Christ's existence and in the Holy Gifts, the Eucharist. When we are partaking of the Eucharist (Greek for "thanksgiving"), we are directly experiencing the mysteries of God, through consumption of Jesus Christ's body and blood. We come into contact with God's ousia, or essence. The body of God is inside our body.*

Listen to the patriarch's words again: "We come into contact with the divine life itself, the very life of heaven. Even though we are on earth, we touch the very kingdom of God." This is the mystery and power of the Jesus Prayer, and the ultimate power of the Eucharist, right here, right now. All time and space have been embraced but also transcended *at the same time*. The limited beings that we are become unlimited through prayer, the Cross, the Christian Church, and the Holy Eucharist. The sins we've committed and continue to commit— "sins" being regrettable mistakes that go against divine law—are cleansed and forgiven. We are free to fully exist and to be the individuals that God has made in his likeness and image, because we are united (or "in communion") with God. We are forgiven because of the great sacrifice that the Second Person of God, Jesus Christ, made in giving his life on the Cross for us.

The mysteries of God become tangible in the Holy Trinity: God, Jesus Christ, and the Holy Spirit, three yet one. In the Church, as a community of believers and lovers of God, the Holy Trinity becomes real in the intersection of the Eucharist. All time stands still. All realities become clearer. Everything that God has created is united.

Take a moment to try the Jesus Prayer: "Lord Jesus Christ, Son of God, have mercy on me, a sinner." (The Holy Trinity is all there in this mystical prayer, as Father Lazarus at St. Antony's Monastery in Egypt taught us.) If that wording feels too cumbersome, try the short form: "Lord, have mercy." If God so moves you, try visiting a church. There you will find a community of seekers, believers, and lovers of God; there you just may experience the Holy Mysteries yourself, through the grace of God.

It all starts with prayer, though, specifically the Jesus Prayer—Lord Jesus Christ, Son of God, have mercy on me—and that's what I want to share with you as we come to this momentary conclusion of our journey together.

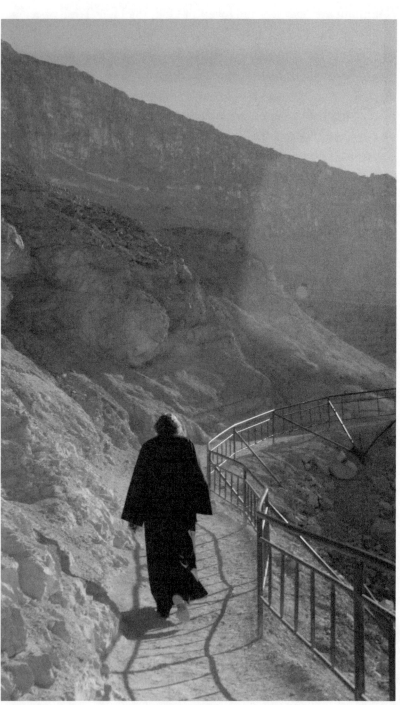

Epilogue

I PRAY THE JESUS PRAYER as much as I can. I'd like to say that I do it constantly, but I haven't quite reached that level yet. I'm working on it. I start my morning, first thing upon waking, with "Thank you, God." Then I begin, "Lord Jesus Christ, Son of God, have mercy on me, a sinner." I say it out loud, but often in a whisper so as not to disturb my wife next to me in bed. Then I say it again. Every so often, about every ten times, I'll replace the phrase "have mercy on me, a sinner" with "thank you, thank you, thank you." I say the prayer when I get up and take some steps. I say it while making coffee, and over breakfast. After awhile, it becomes automatic; that's when I begin to feel a connection with God. Sometimes I catch myself unconsciously saying it—in other words, saying it without realizing that I am. That tells me that it's getting deep inside my soul—or *nous,* as the Greeks say, as Abbot Ephraim at Vatopedi on Mount Athos taught me. This prayer has changed my whole life.

Thinking back over the almost eight years that I've devoted to this project, all I can see is love. It began when Father John and I first had the idea to travel together and make a film and write this book about our experiences. I cherish and am humbled by the outpouring of love

Opposite: Father John Anthony McGuckin ascends the many steps to visit the former cave home of his namesake, St. Antony, on Al-Qalzam Mountain near the Red Sea, Egypt.

from the almost 100 people who have been involved in the logistics, planning, production, translation, writing, editing, and fund-raising that were essential in getting these words to you. The love and kindness that we have received from the almost 100 monks and nuns, abbots, abbesses, superiors, bishops, archbishops, and patriarchs has been profoundly moving for me. For the first time, these men and women who left the world behind in order to be alone with God agreed to share their love, prayers, and practices in a book and on film. As kind and elderly Father Serafim of St. Ana's Monastery in Romania put it, "We the monks have gotten out of the world, but we live here for the sake of the world." They give so much more to us than we give to them.

. . .

Meeting actual hermits, monks, and nuns was at first a little scary. I didn't know what to expect. In hindsight, I realize that I had taken with me a lot of prejudices and assumptions as to what someone who was cloistered might be like. I thought I would encounter real "odd-

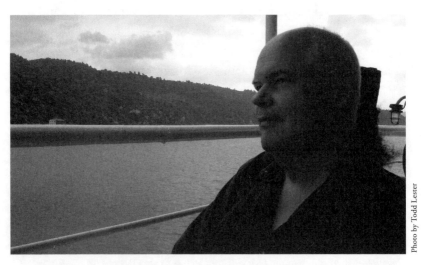

Norris Chumley on the ferry to Mount Athos.

balls." I was expecting highly eccentric people who probably would not want to come near us, much less speak with us. In spite of all the advance permissions we acquired—the years of effort to cut through red tape, the appeals to the highest, most powerful people in church and monastic administrations for help—there was no guarantee whatsoever that any actual monk, hermit, or nun would agree to be interviewed. In reality, I was warned a few times not to take even still cameras to a few monasteries, as we would be turned away.

Yet once we arrived, we were greeted warmly. All my prejudices and anxieties instantly fell away. The monks and nuns were very kind and loving in every respect. Most did not speak English, but they took care to find translators who could assist us. We progressed slowly, spending several days at each location to gain the monks' trust. Of course, most monasteries have visitors (they're called "pilgrims"), and some have even permitted film crews inside the monastery walls in the past, but we were told everywhere we went that no producer or camera crew had *ever* asked the monks and nuns about their souls, let alone what it meant to pray unceasingly, or what it meant to practice the prayer of the heart, the Jesus Prayer. Surprisingly, once I got to know the monks and nuns, I discovered that they were genuinely happy that we had come to inquire about what is most important to them: connection with God. That is what Father Ruwais of St. Antony's Monastery taught us, that prayer is connection with God.

All of the monks and nuns have a lightness of being, a kind of joy-ful zest for life. Some of the monks are just plain funny. As I quoted earlier, Father Jonas, the abbot of St. Jonas Monastery in Kiev, told us, "Without prayer, a monk is just a man in a black dress." His Emi-nence Archbishop Damianos also revealed a sense of humor: after he had outlined the importance of discipline and obedience in prayer and the vital importance of attending all church services on time, he said, "I of course am slothful and many times do not join the fathers in the early morning service!"

· · ·

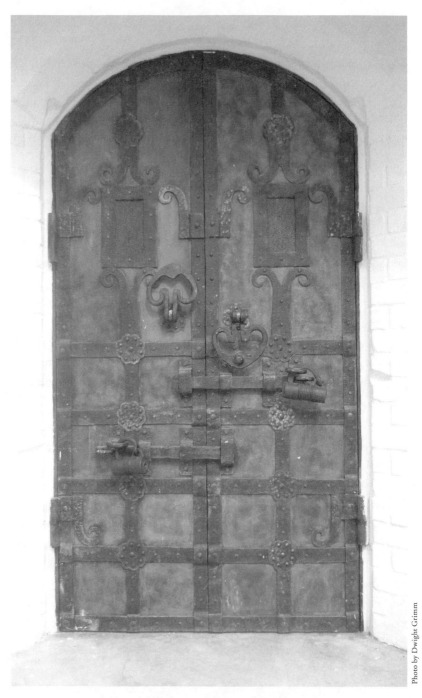

Chapel doorway, Sergiyev Posad Monastery.

Epilogue

The ascetics we met offered a wide range of different descriptions of what it's like to be connected to God, many of which I quoted in an earlier context. For example, Sister Angelina of Pokrovsky Monastery in Kiev said, "God is love, God is quietness, God is peace; and if I feel love and peace in my heart, I know that I am close to God." But consider what Father Lazarus of St. Antony's Monastery in Egypt said, in practical terms: "The truest spiritual life is not permanent peace with calm and no worries. This can be a state of delusion. The truest spiritual life, the best spiritual life, is one when there are these moments of peace. The Lord grants them because he loves us. But a lot of the time we struggle, we fight." Sister Irina mentioned her namesake, St. Irina, whose name means "peace" yet whose death as a martyr was just the opposite. Did Father Lazarus and Sister Irina mean that when we are restless, when we are struggling and fighting and trying to regain our peace, we are not with God?

What I learned from my studies and travels is that at our innermost core, the point where our soul resides, we are always with God, and there exists true peace. The soul is always there, peaceful, uncorrupted. However, it is in our outer layers, our actions and thoughts, where it is often possible to lose connection with God, or perhaps to think or fear that we've lost that precious connection. As Archbishop Justinian in Romania said, "We don't commit sin with our soul. It stays clean and pure." The point is to try to maintain connection with God at all times, remembering that God is here with us at every moment. The practice of prayer and meditation helps us do that, uniting the inner core of our being, our soul, with God and with all the scattered parts of us. His Eminence Archbishop Damianos of St. Catherine's Monastery on Mount Sinai taught us, "There is an icon of God in every single person on earth; and as the Holy Fathers would say, it's the *spermatikos Logos* (the original Word of God). Inside the soul of every person there remains a remembrance of the Creator God the Father."

The point of the Jesus Prayer is to bring soul and body, mind and heart together, in constant remembrance of God in us. In the words of Father Teofil of Romania, its purpose is "to make a link between

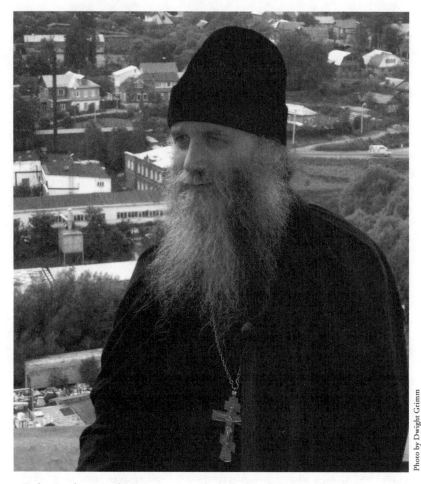

Father Jacob recites the Jesus Prayer in the bell tower at Sergiyev Posad Monastery.

prayer and mind, between mind and heart, between the power that thinks and the power that loves. So the mind that descends its awareness into the heart is not an activity of the human being, it is a work of God. What we are doing is that we pray to God for the unity of our own being, the whole being."

Father Teofil went on to say, "In the gospel we say that God is our Father. This is a God who loves us, a God who is himself love. When God himself settles into our being, he makes a house for himself in our heart. He's hugging us."

Epilogue

Another monk aglow with the love of God is Father Serafim of the Monastery of St. Ana, who put it this way: "Prayer is the breath of the heart. It is the mouth of heaven, of paradise. It is the mouth of the angels. When we pray, we are actually similar to the angels, who are in a state of ceaseless praise for God." He said off-camera that everything around us is speaking of God—nature, the good order of the universe . . . especially other people. *All creation* speaks of God. When we pray the Jesus Prayer, we begin to see God in everything and everyone. This is why, he said, it is important to pray unceasingly, as the angels do: so that we can be reminded of the presence of God everywhere, in everything.

I remember fondly what His Beatitude Patriarch Daniel of Romania said: that we can "discover the icon of Christ in the fellow suffering of others." As I make my way through each day, I struggle with and occasionally suffer from my errors and turbulent thoughts, despite my desire to do well and to be good. Praying the Jesus Prayer frees me up and reminds me of God, especially when I become wrapped up in troubles or am overwhelmed by desires or negativity. I'm shown repeatedly the mercy of God through the person of Christ, and I am again reminded that I am not alone. Struggles cease and my pain is relieved; or, to paraphrase Christ, my yoke is made easy and my burden light.

Father Paisij, monk and deacon of St. Jonas Monastery, urged us to see God in our work. Right after he prayed the Jesus Prayer with us in his cell in Kiev, he said that it is in his study of scripture and the words and teachings of the Holy Fathers and Mothers that God speaks to him. God gives him strength and constant help to get his work done.

The powerful combination of prayer and work is true of Abbess Josephina's vocation as well. In the glorious and creative workshops at Văratec Monastery, we saw Sister Josephina and the nuns unite silence with prayer and work with action. Abbess Josephina taught us to be immersed in prayer always, while completing all physical work that needs to be done. She reminded us of St. Antony, who taught us that one cannot have a life consisting only of prayer; we must use prayer in conjunction with what is necessary to earn a living, and to help

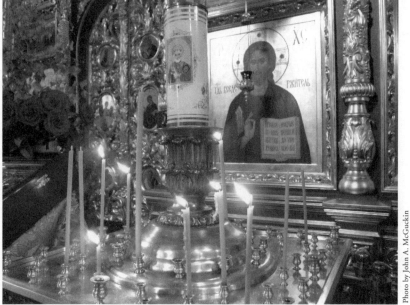

Photo by John A. McGuckin

Icon of Christ Pantocrator, Assumption Cathedral, Sergiyev Posad Monastery, during
the Feast of the Holy Trinity. Note the influence of the ancient Christ Pantocrator
that we saw at St. Catherine's Monastery at Mount Sinai (pictured earlier).

others. When we pray, said the abbess, we feel the love of God, in the
same way that as children we felt the love from our parents when they
held us in their arms.

. . .

At the opening to the monks' caves at the Pecherskaya Lavra in Kiev,
Ukraine, Father Cyril Hovorun said with a giant smile on his face,
"It's a nice image, that the Jesus Prayer initially was practiced in the
caves, and now it can be practiced in the modern caves of people living in blocks in apartments in the megalopolises, in the big cities,
being busy, having everyday heavy duties—but having also reserved
some private space in their hearts and in their minds for the Jesus
Prayer."

Epilogue

Elder Pavlos, the *geron* (or spiritual father—literally "old man") at St. Catherine's, put it very well: "The Jesus Prayer is like a lullaby for the monastics as well as the secular people; it is the nicest thing which exists on earth, this prayer, because it's easy and it revolves around the name of Christ. And when the person gets used to it, he can say it anywhere."

Archbishop Justinian taught us, "When we are in the midst of the Jesus Prayer, we are in the midst of God. We are in the person of God; we see with our eyes, but we don't see him, we feel his presence. We are in his midst." How might you go about this? The loving archbishop told us exactly what he tells his novices:

"Start with the first step; start only with the mouth first—Lord Jesus Christ, Son of God, have mercy upon me—and say it ceaselessly when you go to work or to the office or when you drive. Say this until it becomes a habit; then stop stating it and start doing it silently, only in your thoughts."

The archbishop explained why this works: "When the thoughts feel this, the mouth has no need to issue or utter. . . . The thoughts themselves become a prayer. All alien thoughts are set aside. The mind is no longer concerned with the daily occupations. Now you start having pure thoughts, and pure thoughts exercise a tendency toward the heart and start changing the heart. This is the mystery. This is the sacrament. With this one can get to the illumination."

In the final moments of our journey, at the top of the high bell tower at Sergiyev Posad Monastery in faraway Russia, Father Jacob put this attempt to experience the power of the Jesus Prayer into perspective:

"There is no difference between monastic life and other people," he said. "We have known the circumstances of connection with the world—we left them—and we are free from this world, but nevertheless the love is the same . . . the way to our heavenly father in the love of Jesus Christ, his beloved Son, who became sacrificed for our salvation, is the same. . . . We realize that in the next hour I can die, but my heart, my feelings, my soul, my body, my brains—they belong to

Christ. That's why I'm not afraid of the circumstances of this world—of temptations, of sorrows, of difficulties. . . . We are free with God."

In that place, suffused with the past but invisibly linked with eternity, we prayed the Jesus Prayer together. I held the *lestovka,* the little leather prayer rope, in my hand as I whispered the words in connection with Father John, with Father Jacob, and with God. First in words, then in silence: "Lord Jesus Christ, Son of God, have mercy on me, a sinner."

Acknowledgments

Acknowledgment of Thomas Craughwell

I wish to acknowledge and publicly appreciate my colleague in this book, Thomas Craughwell. Tom is a highly accomplished author and editor, having written such bestsellers as *Saints Behaving Badly* and *Stealing Lincoln's Body*. For many years he was a copywriter for Book-of-the-Month Club. He has been self-employed as an author and editor since 1992.

For the past two years, Tom and I have worked on this book together, and we have become friends in the process. When I first met him, I could tell not only that he had a brilliant mind but also that he was a lot of fun. I might go so far as to say I felt the love of God and Christ in his presence. Needless to say, he has been the perfect collaborator for this project.

Tom's contributions have been enormous. When I gave him volumes of my writings on Christian history, icons, and monasticism, he deftly distilled them into clear and concise prose for general audiences. Meeting with me for interviews and almost endless travel stories, combing through my multiple chapters of reminiscing, Tom helped me bring this book to life.

Acknowledgments

A project of this size, with so many angles and perspectives (such as a feature film, a television special, and multiple Web sites) involves many talents. That he could access every one of them to shape the book you now hold in your hands is evidence of Thomas Craughwell's abilities and deeply held faith.

General Acknowledgments

Above all, I thank God for my life, my family, my interests, and my work. I thank God for love: his love, and my ability to love others and to be loved. I thank God for Jesus Christ, God in a human life, for his teachings and his gift of his life for us. I thank God for the reality of the Cross, for Jesus's resurrection, for the Holy Spirit, and for the Holy Theotokos, the Mother of God incarnate. These are among the Holy Mysteries—with us, for us, in us.

This book, *Mysteries of the Jesus Prayer,* is one of many connected projects arising out of my return to school, with the desire to learn the history of the Christian Church and observe the wondrous disciplines of ascetic life. As I made my way through textbooks and histories, I realized that the only way for me to begin to understand the Holy Mysteries of Christ, and of his gifts in prayer, was to visit the hermits, monks, and nuns and seek a word. I feel so very fortunate and blessed to have had their agreement to appear in this book and film; likewise, I am grateful for their counsel and wisdom, and for the opportunity to share their perspective with others through these projects.

These pursuits are all necessarily done with the companionship and collaboration of a great many people. A few years ago I enrolled in graduate school at Union Theological Seminary in the City of New York for a master of arts degree, then a master of philosophy and eventually a doctor of philosophy degree in theology and the arts, an interdisciplinary program. Very Rev. Dr. John A. McGuckin has been my church history professor and partner in all of the *Mysteries of the Jesus Prayer* projects, and a personal friend as well. I am most grateful to him for encouraging me to write and produce this work. Dr. Janet R. Walton has been my advocate through my scholarly studies and integration of them into artistic expression, and I am most grateful to her as well.

My wife, Catherine Stine Chumley, and sons, Jack Hudson Morris Chumley and Nathaniel Buskirk Chumley, have been loving, tolerant, and encouraging for the last ten years of these works. Many other relatives—my sister, Ellen Chumley, and brothers Hays Chumley, and Gary Buskirk Chumley, sister-in-law Beth Baxter, brother-in-law Neal Baxter, nephew Ross Chumley, brother-in-law John Bower Stine III, sister-in-law Karen Heath Stine, sister-in-law Kanta Bosniak, brother-in-law Richard Laudenslager, Joshua Bosniak, and Murray Bosniak—all mean a great deal to me, and I love them dearly for all of their encouragement. My aunt, Edna Chumley Henderson, has always been one of my biggest fans. Richard Dengler Stine, and Dorothy Cornog Stine, my father-in-law and mother-in-law, and cousins Kathy Funk Arpin and Cindy Funk Carlson and their husbands Donald and Russell, have been avid supporters all along. I thank my parents, Norris Gary Chumley and Mary Ellen Buskirk Chumley, and my grandparents, Hays Hardesty Buskirk, Ruth White Buskirk, Lon Downing Chumley, and Ellen Gary Chumley, and all my ancestors. I say the Jesus Prayer for each of them, with great gratitude.

Aliki Barnstone has been a lifelong friend and exemplar in my studies and in these projects, as has her father, Willis Barnstone, and mother, Helle Tzalopoulou-Barnstone. I would also like to acknowledge lifelong friends Scott Alber and Barbara Hatton Alber, Ruth Hatton Alber and Ruth and Donn Alber, Rob Oudendijk and Yuka Hayashi, Frank and Elaine Haney, Paul and Glenna Pack, David Mallery, Bob and Margery Davis, Curtis and Julie Davis, Fred "Tate" Billings, Michael White, and Kathy and Alan Bremer.

The advisory board for *Mysteries of the Jesus Prayer* has been terrifically helpful in many ways: Macky Alston, Rev. Robert Edgar, Rev. Dr. James A. Forbes Jr., Rev. Dr. Joseph Hough Jr., Harville Hendrix, Helen LaKelly Hunt, Judith D. Moyers, James A. Sanders, Rev. Dr. Robert and Nikki Stephanopoulos, and Robert Thurman, Bill Moyers has also been great, as have Sandy Heberer and Cara Liebenson. My doctoral board has been invaluable to my Christian education

Acknowledgments

and mission to help others: Euan K. Cameron, Rev. John Chryssav-gis, and George C. Stoney. Todd Edison French and David Sanchez have been my doctoral fellows and friends. Scott Cairns has been a spiritual brother and friend. Rev. Dr. Michael Kinnamon, Antonios Kireopoulos, and Pat Pattilo at the National Council of Churches of Christ helped us "get the Word out."

Our funders for the documentary feature film *Mysteries of the Jesus Prayer* played a vital role. Our major donors and bellwethers the Virginia H. Farah Foundation, the Avalon Foundation, Harville Hendrix, Helen LaKelly Hunt, Abby and Stephen Wise, Arthur Trotman, Nancy Fish, Mary Reilly, Charles and Pam Perkins, Marcus Pauls, Lucas Pauls, Sandra Kress, Anne Jarrell, Judith and Jerry Miller, Derek Berg and Janice Ellsworth, Michael and Cynthia Schlegel, Marian Warden, Darelyn Olsen, Susan Hermanson, Jim Selfe, the Brauner Foundation, Calvin Mew, Susan Schulte Braddock, and Aldon James are like earthly angels. I thank the board and members of the National Arts Club for hosting a benefit for the film. The Hart-ley Film Foundation has been our fiscal sponsor and I thank their board, Sarah Masters and Laura Healy.

I am deeply thankful to His All Holiness Bartholomew I, Arch-bishop of Constantinople, New Rome, and Ecumenical Patriarch, for his foreword and overall support and assistance.

There are several people from the Orthodox Churches and the monasteries that have been immeasurably helpful; I list them in chronological sequence of their assistance to the project. His Eminence Archbishop Demetrios of America; His Holiness Pope Shenouda III; His Eminence Archbishop Damianos of Sinai; His Beatitude Patriarch Theoctist, Patriarch of All Romania; His Beati-tude Patriarch Daniel, Patriarch of All Romania, and His Eminence Kirill, Patriarch of Moscow and All Russia. Additionally, many abbots and abbesses and heads of Orthodox Church external affairs offices have been extraordinarily helpful. I thank them for permission to film in the monasteries and for introducing us to the monks and nuns, and for their participation and wise instruction: Abbot Ephraim of Vatopedi, Father Makarios of Taxiarches, His Grace Bishop Yustus of

Acknowledgments

St. Antony's, His Eminence Bishop Youannes of Cairo, His Eminence Laurenţiu Streza of Sâmbăta de Sus, His Eminence Iustin Sigheteanul of St. Ana, His Eminence Justinian Chira Maramureşeanul, Sister Irina Pântescu of Voroneţ, Sister Josephina Giosanu of Văratec, Rev. Prof. Ioan Mihoc, Sister Olimpiada Chiriac, Archimandrite Clement Haralam, Father Cyril Hovorun of the Pecherskaya Lavra, Archimandrite Jonas of St. Jonas Monastery, Archbishop Feognost of Sergiyev Posad, and Father George Kirindas of the Moscow Patriarchate. Father Alexander Karloutsos and Rev. Father Mark Arey have been wonderfully helpful. We have been blessed with some wonderful guides, logistical and spiritual, at the monasteries: Father Ruwais, Father Lazarus, Father Justin, Father Gregory, Elder Pavlos, Archimandrite Serafim Man, Rev. Dan Sandu, Father Dorinel Dani, Deacon Anthony and Helen Vovchenko, and Zinoviy Chesnokov. I thank the monks and nuns—Father Neilos, Father Gregory, Father Daniel, Archimandrite Teofil, Mother Maria, Father Paisij, Father Maxim, Sister Galena, Sister Angelina, and Father Jacob—for so generously appearing in the film and for their interviews.

There have been seven languages in use in this project, and our translators have been essential: Helle Tzalopoulou-Barnstone, Rev. George Zugravu, Rev. Dan Sandu, Fevronia K. Soumakis, Aheb Kamel, Sophronies Michaelides, Sergey Trostianskiy, and Zinoviy Chesnokov. C. Paul Grenier has been a marvelous transcriber. All of our interviews were conducted with a translator to interpret both our questions and the interviewees' responses as needed. After these taped interviews were transcribed, the translators then edited the English version for translational accuracy.

I thank my agent, John Thornton, and HarperOne publisher, Mark Tauber, and Roger Freet, my editor, for bringing this book to life. Hugh Van Dusen has been a trusted friend over the years. Steven Waldman and Elizabeth Sams of Beliefnet have supported my ideas all along. Todd Lester has been a helpful friend and field associate producer.

I am delighted to share the artistic work of iconographer Eileen McGuckin and appreciate her overall support of these projects.

Acknowledgments

Many photographs in this book are by her husband, Father John A. McGuckin, and our cinematographers, Patrick Gallo, Dwight Grimm, and John Foster. I thank David Aslan, our documentary feature film editor and producer; Richard Devletian, our sound designer and composer; Chao-Ying Lin, our website designer; and Taili Wu, our digital art director and animations designer. We've had excellent interns working with us on postproduction: Sarah Sellman, Alex Forstenhausler, and Yunah Chung.

We are grateful for the assistance of the Egyptian Mission to the United Nations Press Office, Ismail Khairat and Rosanna and Mrs. Mahmoud Basma; the Romanian Tourist Office, Simion Alb; the Romanian Cultural Institute, Corina Suteu; Consulate General of Ukraine in New York, Bohdan Movchan; Enjoy Travel in Egypt, Ahmed Said; Central Hotel in Ploeşti, Romania; Sky Gate Golden Tulip, Bucharest-Otopeni, Romania; American Business Center in Ukraine, Igor Issayev; Restaurant Khutorets in Kyiv, Ukraine, and Royal Card Restaurants, Ukraine.

Finally, there are lots of friends, colleagues, and allies who have helped launch this book and myriad projects in unique ways: Jesse Willmon, Kirsten Sorton, Donald Kautz, Bowie Snodgrass, George Matthew, Elizabeth Harding, John Snodgrass, Justin Lasser, Mark C. Taylor, Alfred Stepan, Emily Brennan, His Eminence Archbishop Nicholae Condrea, Anton C. Vrame, Patton Burchett, Dan and Julia Vaca, Spyros and Katerina Tsimouris, Rev. Vasileos Thermos, Leila A. Bakry-Becker, Alejandra Trillos, Hugo Espinel, Alexandra Zobel, Ashley J. French, Bethany Cole, Craig Cones, Zoe Barnstone Clark, Neil Sharrow, Polly Campbell, Monique van Kerkhof, Lou Volpicelli, Eileen Newman, Dan Coughlin, and Al Cattabiani.

Suggested Reading

Anonymous. *The Way of a Pilgrim and the Pilgrim Continues His Way.* Translated by R. M. French. San Francisco: HarperOne, 1991.

The Apostolic Fathers. Second ed. Translated by J. B. Lightfoot and J. R. Harmer. Grand Rapids, MI: Baker Book House, 1992.

The Art of Prayer: An Orthodox Anthology. Compiled by Igumen Chariton of Valamo. Translated by E. Kadloubovsky and E. M. Palmer. Edited with a foreword by Timothy Ware. London: Faber and Faber, 1997.

Athanasius. *The Life of Antony.* Translated by Tim Vivian, Apostolos N. Athanassakis, John Serapion, Rowan A. Greer, and Benedicta Ward. Cistercian Studies Series. Kalamazoo, MI: Cistercian Publications, 2003.

Augustine. "Letter 130: To Proba." Father of the Church. www.newadvent.org/fathers/1102.htm.

His All Holiness Ecumenical Patriarch Bartholomew. *Encountering the Mystery: Understanding Orthodox Christianity Today.* New York: Doubleday, 2008.

———. *In the World, Yet Not of the World: Social and Global Initiatives of Ecumenical Patriarch Bartholomew.* Bronx, NY: Fordham University Press, 2010.

Brianchaninov, Ignatius, with a foreword by Kallistos Ware. *On the Prayer of Jesus.* Boston: New Seeds Books, 2006.

Chryssavgis, John, and Abba Zosimas. *In the Heart of the Desert: The Spirituality of the Desert Fathers and Mothers—With a Translation of Abba Zosimas' Reflections.* Treasures of the World's Religions. Bloomington, IN: World Wisdom, 2003.

Ciobotea, Daniel (metropolitan and patriarch). *Confessing the Truth in Love: Orthodox Perceptions on Life, Mission, and Unity.* Iaşi, Romania: Trinitas, 2001.

Climacus, John. *The Ladder of Divine Ascent.* Translated by Colm Luibhéid and Norman Russell. Classics of Western Spirituality. Mahwah, NJ: Paulist Press, 1982.

Dalrymple, William. *From the Holy Mountain: A Journey in the Shadow of Byzantium.* London: HarperCollins, 1997.

Suggested Reading

Gillet, Lev (archimandrite). *The Jesus Prayer.* Edited and with a foreword by Kallistos Ware. Crestwood, NY: St. Vladimir's Seminary Press, 1987. Original French version, 1963, published pseudonymously by "A monk of the Eastern Church."

Harmless, William. *Desert Christians: An Introduction to the Literature of Early Monasticism.* London: Oxford Univ. Press, 2004.

John of the Cross. *The Collected Works of St. John of the Cross.* Vol. II. Translated by David Lewis. New York: Cosimo, 2007.

Louth, Andrew. *The Wilderness of God.* London: Darton, Longman and Todd, 1991.

Mathewes-Green, Frederica. *The Jesus Prayer: The Ancient Desert Prayer That Tunes the Heart to God.* Orleans, MA: Paraclete Press, 2009.

McGuckin, John Anthony. *At the Lighting of the Lamps: Hymns of the Ancient Church.* Oxford, UK: SLG Press, 1995.

———. *The Book of Mystical Chapters: Meditations on the Soul's Ascent from the Desert Fathers and Other Early Christian Contemplatives.* Boston: Shambhala, 2002.

———. *Standing in God's Holy Fire: The Byzantine Tradition.* London: Darton, Longman and Todd, 2001.

Moschos, John. *The Spiritual Meadow (Pratum Spirituale).* Translated by John Wortley. Kalamazoo, MI: Cistercian Publications, 1992.

Philokalia, The. Volumes 1-5. Translated by G.E.H. Palmer, Philip Sherrard, and Kallistos Ware. London: Faber and Faber, 1995.

Salinger, J. D. *Franny and Zooey.* New York: Back Bay Books, 2001.

A Selected Library of Nicene and Post-Nicene Fathers of the Christian Church, second series. Volume 10: St. Ambrose, Selected Works and Letters. Translated by Philip Schaff and Henry Wace. London: Parker & Company, 1896.

Sherrard, Philip. *Athos, the Mountain of Silence.* London, New York: Oxford Univ. Press, 1960.

Spencer, Matthew. *Athos: Travels on the Holy Mountain.* London: Azure, 2000.

Ward, Benedicta. *The Wisdom of the Desert Fathers: The Apophthegmata Patrum (the Anonymous Series).* Oxford, UK: SLG Press, 1975.

———. *The Sayings of the Desert Fathers: The Alphabetical Collection.* Kalamazoo, MI: Cistercian Publications, 1984.

Ware, Kallistos. *The Orthodox Way.* Rev. ed. Crestwood, NY: St. Vladimir's Seminary Press, 1998.

———. *The Power of the Name: The Jesus Prayer in Orthodox Spirituality.* Oxford, UK: SLG Press, 1974.

Williams, Charles, ed. *The Letters of Evelyn Underhill.* London: Longmans, Green and Co., 1943.

Index

Index

Index

Index

Index

Index

Index

For the *Mysteries of the Jesus Prayer* feature film,
free newsletters, study guides, transcripts, chants,
and prayers, please visit our website

www.JesusPrayerMovie.com